Procedures in Practice

Procedures
in Practice

Published by the British Medical Journal
Tavistock Square, London WC1H 9JR

First edition 1981
Second edition 1988
Reprinted 1989
Reprinted 1991

British Library Cataloguing in Publication Data

Procedures in practice.
1. Medicine. Techniques
1. British Medical Journal
610′.28
ISBN 0–7279–0218–0

Typeset in Great Britain by
Latimer Trend & Company Ltd, Plymouth
Printed in Great Britain at the
University Press, Cambridge

Contents

Arterial puncture

D C FLENLEY

Introduction

Arterial puncture is carried out in order to measure the arterial blood gas tensions (Pao_2 and $Paco_2$), oxygen saturation (Sao_2), and pH (or $[H^+]$) so as to determine (1) abnormalities in the gas exchanging function of the lungs, for which it is necessary to know also the concentration of oxygen being inspired at the time of puncture; and (2) the patient's acid base state, by relating the $Paco_2$ to the pH (or $[H^+]$), both to diagnose a disorder and as a guide to its treatment.

Indications

Arterial puncture is thus essential for the accurate diagnosis of respiratory failure, which may have been suspected clinically by noting central cyanosis. Only by knowing arterial blood gas tensions can the type of respiratory failure be identified—for example, type I with a low Po_2 and normal or low Pco_2; or type II, in which a low Po_2 is associated with a high Pco_2. As the management of these two conditions may differ considerably, accurate diagnosis is essential.

Although measurement of the venous bicarbonate concentration will give some indication of the severity of a *metabolic* acid base disturbance, definition of the type and severity of a *respiratory* acid base disturbance can be made only when arterial Pco_2 and pH (or $[H^+]$) are known.

Contraindications

Contraindications to arterial puncture include a bleeding diathesis, as, for example, a platelet count below $30 \times 10^9/l$; and disturbance of clotting factors as in haemophilia and hypoprothrombinaemia or after overdoses of anticoagulants such as heparin, etc. In these conditions arterial puncture may lead to an excessive local haematoma, and this may also rarely complicate arterial puncture in patients with a diastolic blood pressure over 120 mm Hg.

Site of puncture

The brachial artery, just above the elbow crease, of the non-dominant arm—that is, the left arm in a right handed

1

person—is preferred. Patients are used to blood sampling at this site, where the artery is usually easily palpated, and personal experience shows that a small haematoma in the antecubital fossa is not painful, in contrast to a similar sized haematoma after puncture of the radial artery at the wrist. Puncture of the femoral artery in the groin is not advised, as this site is embarrassing to the patient, inconvenient for the operator, and not infrequently yields blood from the femoral vein, which is much larger than the accompanying femoral artery—an error that can lead to potentially grave mistakes in diagnosis and treatment.

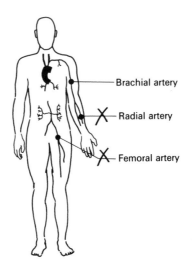

Equipment

- Equipment for skin preparation (swabs, 1% cetrimide, etc).
- Some 1% plain lignocaine (without adrenaline) contained in a 5 ml syringe fitted with an orange (25 G) needle for local anaesthesia. This is *always* required: anyone who doubts this should be subjected to arterial puncture without it! The arterial puncture is carried out with a sterile *all glass, heavily siliconised 10 ml syringe*, in which the barrel moves easily. This syringe contains a stainless steel washer, and the dead space is filled with a solution of heparin containing 1000 U/ml. The syringe is fitted with a green (21 G) disposable needle with a conventional bevel.

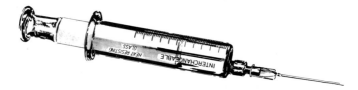

- Two or three 7·5 cm gauze swabs, and a 7·5 cm crepe bandage.

Before you start

Clearly, you will explain to the patient what you are about to do. Emphasise that you are going to use local anaesthetic and that he will feel the "jag" of the injection, but should not thereafter feel the actual arterial puncture. It is important to check that the plunger of the all glass syringe slides easily with minimal resistance when suction is applied, so that the arterial blood will flush into the syringe spontaneously. Do not forget to fill the dead space (the syringe and the needle) with a heparin solution of 1000 U/ml strength before using it. It also helps to let the heparin solution wet the walls of the syringe by sucking a little heparin into the syringe, then moving the plunger down, and finally expelling any remaining air bubble by holding the syringe vertically with the needle uppermost.

Make sure that if the patient is breathing oxygen the method by which this is given, and the flow rate (for example, nasal prongs: 2 l oxygen/min), is noted on the laboratory request form, and that the flow rate has not been changed for at least 15 minutes before the arterial puncture is carried out. This is to avoid any likelihood of changes in arterial oxygen tension (Po_2) arising from poor equilibration within the lungs, which can occur in patients with lung disease and ventilation perfusion imbalance for several minutes after a change in the inspired oxygen concentration. It is also useful to state on the laboratory request form that the patient was breathing air, and not merely leave the laboratory staff to guess that that was the case because no oxygen administration was stated.

Procedure

Outpatients should be seated, and the left arm may easily be supported on the edge of the consulting desk, to hyperextend the arm at the elbow. In patients in bed the arm may be hyperextended on a pillow. It is essential to make sure that the brachial artery can be palpated, the artery usually lying slightly medial to the tendon of the biceps at the top of the antecubital fossa. After skin preparation 0·5–1·0 ml of the local anaesthetic is infiltrated on each side of the artery and then, as the needle is withdrawn, a small bleb left just under the skin. To prevent injection of lignocaine into the artery it is advisable always to attempt to withdraw fluid into the syringe before injecting at any site. If this withdrawal yields bloodstaining the needle point should be moved before the local anaesthetic is injected.

The patient should be warned that he may have some tingling and numbness in the hand, which may last for 30–60 minutes after puncture, but that this results from partial anaesthesia of the median nerve, which lies very close to the brachial artery in the antecubital fossa. This symptom is of no clinical consequence.

After leaving two to three minutes for the local anaesthetic to act use the arterial puncture syringe, with a green (21 G)

3

3·8 cm (1·5 in) needle attached, to obtain the sample of arterial blood. With the bevel upwards the needle is advanced through the skin bleb of local anaesthetic towards the pulsations of the brachial artery, which is continuously palpated by two fingers of the operator's left hand. The syringe is held with the needle at some 30° or so to the skin surface and is advanced proximally almost to touch the surface of the humerus. The syringe is then steadily withdrawn while slight suction is maintained on the plunger. At some point blood will suddenly enter the syringe, when suction and movement of the syringe should cease. With the syringe held still the blood must be seen to *pulsate into the syringe under its own power*. This is the only proof of successful arterial puncture.

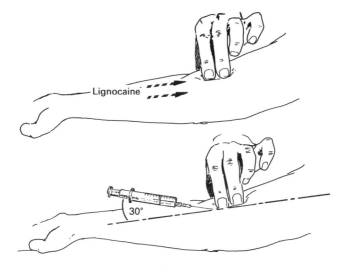

As arterial puncture is usually carried out in patients with central cyanosis, in whom even arterial blood will appear bluish, the colour of the blood is never a reliable indicator that arterial, and not venous, blood is being sampled. Without moving the syringe gentle suction is then continued until a 5–6 ml sample is obtained, but suction should then again cease to reaffirm that blood is still pulsating into the syringe.

Aftercare

A folded 7·5 cm gauze swab is then firmly applied with the left hand over the puncture site and the needle and arterial puncture syringe completely withdrawn. The syringe is laid aside and firm pressure maintained over the puncture site through the gauze swab. This swab is then held firmly in position by a 7·5 cm crepe bandage wrapped around the arm, each turn of the bandage being tightened. This firm bandage pressure, which will usually cause the arm below the bandage to become blue owing to obstruction of venous return, is maintained for five minutes. At the end of this time it is the responsibility of the operator to ensure that the bandage is removed.

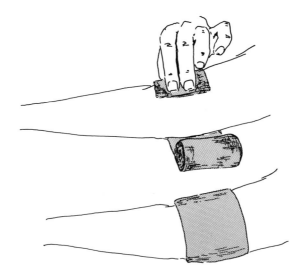

After the bandage has been applied the syringe containing the arterial blood is taken in the right hand, with the plunger supported in the palm to prevent it from falling out. The needle is removed, and the one or two discrete air bubbles (all that are permitted) gently expelled by tapping the side of the syringe and pushing the plunger upwards so as to expel some blood into a swab held over the tip of the syringe. The syringe is then capped and gently inverted two or three times to allow the stainless steel washer within the syringe to mix the sample.

The patient is warned that he may have a small haematoma over the site of puncture the following day. A useful way of expressing this is to say, "You may have a small bruise there tomorrow—if you do you will know that I am an honest doctor, and if you don't you may even think I'm a good one." Most patients appreciate such a comment.

Arterial puncture should be almost painless and thus not provoke hyperventilation due to anxiety or pain, which would tend to lower the Pco_2 and increase pH (lower hydrogen ion concentration), so adding a spurious temporary respiratory alkalosis to any other acid base disturbance.

The specimen

The sample is then taken directly to be injected into the blood gas electrodes from the syringe without transfer to any other container. Blood gas analysis should be carried out within five or not more than 10 minutes of removing the sample from the patient, and the sample should not be cooled during this period. If a greater delay is inevitable cooling the syringe and its contents in ice, with subsequent rewarming to body temperature before analysis, may help to minimise errors caused by continued metabolism of the white cells within the blood sample. This, however, is a compromise that is undesirable in practice, and measurement within five minutes of sampling is much preferred for accurate results.

The syringe must be well lubricated by the heparin solution and have siliconised walls to ensure that the barrel moves easily under the patient's own pulsatile arterial blood pressure. The needle must fit tightly, and only very slight suction is applied, to prevent a froth of air and blood from forming within the syringe, which invalidates the anaerobic sample and makes the measurement meaningless. One or at most two small discrete bubbles are permitted, but these should be promptly expelled after the puncture as described above.

Recently Radiometer introduced a special arterial blood gas sampling syringe (B109), which appears to be a useful method of obtaining a small sample of arterial blood suitable for use with the new automatic microsample blood gas electrode systems. A similar special syringe is made by Concord Laboratories (Pulsator). Nevertheless, I prefer a larger sample, as this allows the measurements to be duplicated on the same sample, thus increasing confidence in the results.

Interpretation of results

To use arterial blood gas analysis to measure any abnormality in the gas exchange function of the lungs it is essential that the approximate concentration of inspired oxygen at the time of withdrawing the arterial sample should be known. For example, with nasal prongs giving 2 l oxygen/min this concentration is about 30%; with the Ventimask (35%, 28%, 24%) the concentration is known more accurately, although most patients tolerate any masks less than the nasal prongs. With high concentration oxygen treatment, as with the Polymask, 6 l oxygen/min delivers about 60% oxygen. At sea level the inspired oxygen tension (PIo_2) is then 60 kPa for 60% inspired oxygen, 30 kPa for 30% inspired oxygen, etc.

The alveolar to arterial oxygen tension gradient ($A\text{-}aDo_2$) can then be estimated at the bedside, assuming that the patient's gas exchange ratio (R) is 1·0–0·8, which is usually true in most clinical circumstances.

Then, approximately,

$$PAo_2 = PIo_2 - \frac{Paco_2}{R}$$

$$A\text{-}aDo_2 = PAo_2 - Pao_2$$

where PAo_2 = calculated value of alveolar oxygen tension, PIo_2 = tension of inspired oxygen, $Paco_2$ = measured value of arterial Pco_2, and Pao_2 = measured value of arterial Po_2. In a normal adult at sea level, breathing air at rest, $A\text{-}aDo_2$ does not exceed 3·5 kPa (26 mm Hg). Normal arterial Pco_2 is 5·0–5·5 kPa (38–41 mm Hg), and arterial Po_2 10–14 kPa (75–105 mm Hg). In respiratory alkalosis the arterial Pco_2 will be below normal whereas the arterial pH will be higher than normal; in respiratory acidosis the arterial Pco_2 will be above normal and the arterial pH lower than normal. Conversely, in metabolic acidosis the arterial Pco_2 will be below normal and the arterial pH will also be below normal, whereas in metabolic alkalosis the arterial P_{CO_2} will tend to be higher than normal and the pH will also be higher than normal.

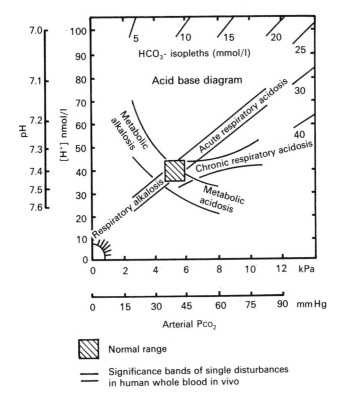

Normal range

Significance bands of single disturbances in human whole blood in vivo

Acid base disturbances can be characterised more exactly by the relations between the measured Pa_{CO_2} (or $[H^+]$) by plotting these values on an acid base diagram, which is based on the empirically observed relations between these variables in the arterial blood of human patients with disease.

The acid base diagram is reproduced from the *British Journal of Hospital Medicine* by kind permission of the editor.

Aspiration and injection of joints

MICHAEL GUMPEL

Introduction

Septic arthritis, diagnosed and treated early, need not lead to irreversible joint damage. Undiagnosed or inadequately treated joint sepsis often leads to irreversible joint damage, which is not amenable to joint replacement. Aspiration of potentially infected joints before use of antibiotics is therefore an important part of the repertoire of every hospital doctor. While some cases of septic arthritis can be diagnosed circumstantially on the basis of positive cultures elsewhere, such as blood or wound swabs, only joint aspiration will give accurate information. Similarly, gout may be diagnosed clinically, but only the identification of intracellular uric acid crystals will give a definitive diagnosis.

In this age of disposable needles and syringes, therapeutic intra-articular and periarticular injections are practicable and mutually satisfying procedures in general practice.

This chapter cannot cover all the detail. If you would like not only to read about the procedures but see them carried out a visit to your friendly local rheumatologist in his clinic will get you started.

Indications and contraindications

The common indications for joint aspiration and for injection are shown in the table. Joints containing prostheses are the province of orthopaedic surgeons. Where sepsis is a possibility corticosteroid injections are contraindicated until negative bacterial cultures have been obtained. Septic joints should be aspirated to "dryness" and aspirated daily until free from effusion. Acute haemarthroses should be fully aspirated also; in most other circumstances this is not necessary. Chronic indolent infection, especially with tuberculosis, is easily missed.

Regularly repeated injections are thought to cause premature damage to the articular cartilage, and the need for repeated injection should be tempered by consideration of other factors—for example, poor muscle, joint instability, or damage requiring expert opinion. In athletes and other patients in whom overuse of joints has occurred, corticosteroid injections should not be considered an easy alternative to rest; in particular, the achilles tendon is prone to rupture, particularly after inexpert injections.

Indications

Joint aspiration	Joint injection
Diagnostic Undiagnosed acute effusion: (a) ? septic (b) ? crystal induced (c) ? traumatic (d) ? haemarthrosis	*Diagnostic* (a) Arthrography — usually double contrast for meniscal tears (b) Arthrography in investigation of calf pain or swelling ? ruptured knee capsule, *or* ? ruptured Baker's cyst
Therapeutic (a) Tense acute effusion (b) Interference with function (c) Septic joint (d) Haemarthrosis	*Therapeutic* (a) Persistent monoarthritis (b) Enthesiopathy — for example, painful shoulder, tennis elbow (c) Improve function — for example, in rheumatoid arthritis (d) Peritendinitis
Contraindications or special care (a) Haemophilia (b) Prosthetic joint	*Contraindications or special care* (a) Infection, acute or chronic (b) Prosthetic joint (c) Repeated corticosteroid injections (d) Athletic or overuse situations (e) Achilles tendon

Equipment

Chlorhexidine in spirit, or Hibiscrub and adequate washing facilities, sterile needles and syringes, and a no touch procedure are all the expert needs. For the less experienced, surgical drapes, gloves, and a sterile surface are important; so is an adequate amount of lignocaine. Saline should be on the trolley: in the event of a "dry" tap, the saline can be used to check free flow into the joint and the washings can go for microbiological examination. Gillette flip top needles are the most convenient.

Single dose ampoules are safest, unless you are the sole or first user of multidose phials. Hydrocortisone acetate is safe, cheap, and usually effective. Methylprednisolone acetate and triamcinolone (hex) acetonide may act for longer but are more likely to cause a post-injection flare and skin atrophy when injected close to the skin.

- A rigorous aseptic no touch procedure
- Chlorhexidine in spirit
- Selection of syringes: 20, 10, 5, 2 ml
- Selection of needles: 19, 21, 23, 25 G (preferably Gillette type of pack)
- Ampoules of local anaesthetic (without adrenaline)
- Ampoules of sterile saline
- Forceps (for jammed needles)

Optional
- Sterile cotton wool balls
- Sterile receiver or jug
- Sterile gloves
- Sterile drapes
- Sticky plasters
- Crepe bandage

For injection
- Hydrocortisone *acetate* ampoules *or*
- Methylprednisolone acetate *or*
- Triamcinolone (hex) acetonide

Containers
- Sterile containers for microbiology, cytology (? + heparin), crystals (? + heparin)
- Lithium container for biochemistry, protein
- Fluoride container for synovial fluid glucose or blood glucose

General procedure

Diagnostic aspiration or injection is much easier when appreciable swelling is present, as less precision is required in placing the needle. Before starting, carefully feel the bony margins of the joint space. Use the thumbnail to mark the joint space, and if in doubt move one bone so that you can feel its movement on one side of the joint. Check that you have easily available all you need: choice of needles and syringes, local anaesthetic (or saline), requisite specimen containers, and, for large effusions, a jug or basin nearby. For aspiration followed by injection draw up the steroid beforehand and make sure the needles are not too tightly jammed on the syringes.

Prepare the skin carefully with chlorhexidine in 5% spirit or surgical spirit—not Savlon. A rigorous no touch technique is for the experienced and for simple injections; sterile gloves, a sterile pack, and a generous area of prepared skin for the less experienced. With experience it is rarely necessary to use local anaesthetic, and a subcutaneous bleb is usually sufficient. Local anaesthetic in the syringe is useful when difficulty in entering the joint is expected or to clear the needle and check that there is free and easy flow once the joint is entered.

In joint aspiration the needle size is important. For thick, purulent, or chronic effusions a white (19 G) needle is usually needed; otherwise a green one (21 G) will suffice. For finger and toe joints use a blue (23 G) needle, which is usually used for injecting small quantities.

When effusions are purulent send specimens for microbiological examination and measurement of protein and glucose concentrations (in a small fluoride container), and a heparinised sample for cytology and crystal examination. Identifying crystals requires some experience, and at night it may be best to keep a sample refrigerated for re-examination next morning.

Knee

The patient should be as comfortable as possible, lying down with sufficient pillows. The knee may be slightly flexed and muscles relaxed. Palpate the posterior edge of the patella medially or laterally and move the patella gently sideways to feel the femoral surfaces below. The patient should be sufficiently relaxed that the patella can be moved freely; otherwise, aspiration is virtually impossible. Maintain a gentle conversation rather than grim silence. Insert the needle horizontally or slightly downwards into the joint in the gap between patella and femur; once behind the patella it must be within the joint. A slight resistance may often be felt as the needle goes through the synovial membrane. If no fluid can be aspirated check that the patient's quadriceps muscle is relaxed and that the needle is not blocked by injecting local anaesthetic. If this flows freely the needle is intra-articular. One last trick is to rotate the needle, as a synovial villus or fibrin body may be against the bevel.

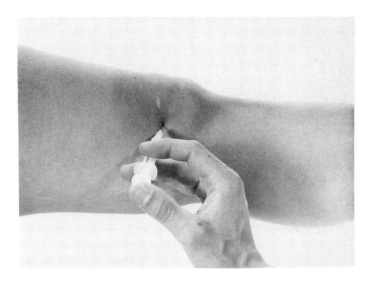

Small effusions may sometimes be found in the medial or lateral pouches, and fluid will appear in the syringe as the needle is withdrawn very slowly with negative pressure. Once the correct position is found, rest the hand holding the syringe against the patient's leg. The usual dose is 50 mg hydrocortisone acetate, 40 mg methylprednisolone, or 20 mg triamcinolone (hex) acetonide. If injecting steroid do not completely aspirate the joint, so as to permit free diffusion of steroid around the cavity.

Prepatella bursitis

Several bursae are present on the lower surface of the patella and patellar tendon. While bursitis will usually respond to using a kneeling pad, some cases are sufficiently painful to warrant injecting 25 mg hydrocortisone acetate into the most tender area.

11

Ankle joint

With the foot slightly plantar flexed, palpate the joint line anteriorly between the tendons of extensor hallucis longus laterally and tibialis anterior medially just above the tip of the medial malleolus. Direct the needle slightly sideways, backwards, and upwards. Fluid may be aspirated if there is an effusion. Hydrocortisone acetate 25 mg is appropriate.

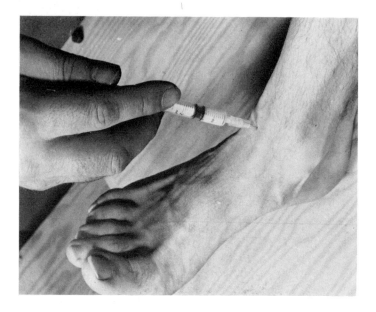

Shoulder

The shoulder joint is most easily entered anteriorly: this route is used for aspiration, frozen shoulder, and synovitis. With the patient seated and his arm relaxed against the side of the chest, feel for the space between the head of the humerus and the glenoid cap, about 1 cm below the coracoid process. If in doubt, rotate the humerus by moving the extended hand outwards and feel the head moving under the fingers. Insert the needle into the space with a slight medial angle. It should enter the joint easily, almost to the length of a green needle. The usual dose is 25–50 mg hydrocortisone acetate.

The lateral approach is used mainly for subacromial bursitis or the painful arc syndrome. Feel for the lateral tip of the acromium and insert the needle just below it in a medial direction with a slight downward slant until the tip reaches the humeral head. Gradually withdraw the needle with gentle pressure on the plunger: when the needle point is in the subacromial bursa a sudden drop in resistance will be felt. Injection will often reproduce the symptoms of the painful arc syndrome; if it does not, angle the needle in different directions until the pain is reproduced. Mixing local anaesthetic with the steroid is a useful diagnostic test, as the shoulder movements (or symptoms) should be improved after a few minutes. A second injection after a few days is often required.

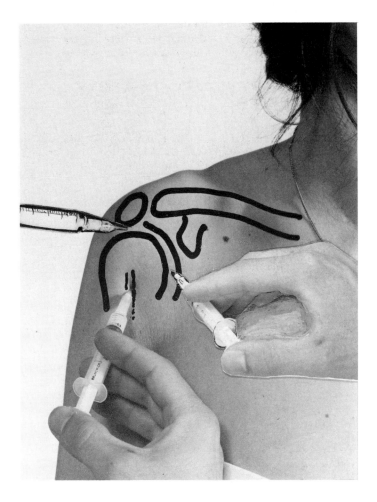

Bicipital tendinitis is one cause of shoulder pain and is detected by finding tenderness over the tendon when the arm is externally rotated. Insert the needle almost parallel to the tendon—if it enters the tendon there will be resistance to the injection—then withdraw slightly and inject 25 mg hydrocortisone acetate into the tendon sheath and 25 mg direct into the shoulder joint, as part of the tendon is intra-articular.

Elbow

Care is needed to differentiate between the possible sites of pain. Tennis and golfer's elbow are the common reasons for injection. The elbow is not an easy joint to inject, except in the presence of an effusion. The lateral approach is just proximal to the radial head, with the elbow flexed at 90°. Palpate the radial head while rotating the patient's hand, and locate the proximal end. Insert the needle between this and

13

the lateral epicondyle at about 90° to the skin. The posterior approach may be used, again with the elbow at 90°, with the needle aimed between the olecranon process and the lateral epicondyle.

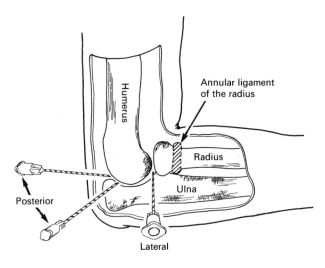

Tennis elbow

Carefully locate the site of maximal pain over the annular ligament of the radius and muscle attachments to it or to the lateral humeral epicondyle. Using a green or blue needle, infiltrate (with considerable pressure) 25 mg hydrocortisone acetate and 1 ml local anaesthetic in and around the area of maximal tenderness, reinserting the needle down to bone in several areas without completely withdrawing it. After some five minutes check that the local tenderness has disappeared. A second injection is often needed after a few days.

Golfer's elbow

Once again, carefully localise the maximal point of tenderness at the insertion of muscles into the medial epicondyle of the humerus and medial ligament, and inject as for tennis elbow. Remember to palpate and avoid the ulnar nerve in the groove below the medial epicondyle.

Wrist

The easiest site for injecting the wrist is just distal to the ulnar head, on the dorsal surface of the wrist and slightly inside (to the radial side). In theory several separate synovial cavities may exist, but in practice, particularly with persistent synovitis, usually all of these interconnect. Carefully palpate the space between the ulnar head and the lunate, and insert the needle at right angles to the skin between the extensor tendons to the ring and little fingers to a depth of about 1·0–1·5 cm. With careful palpation and marking, the needle will slip into a space between bones. The usual dose is 25 mg hydrocortisone acetate.

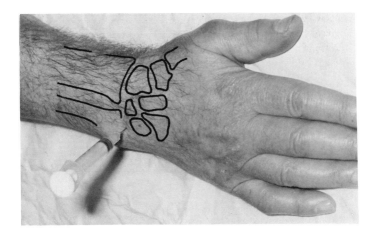

De Quervain's tenosynovitis

Tenosynovitis may occur in synovial sheaths surrounding the tendons of extensor pollicis longus and occasionally abductor pollicis longus as they pass through the extensor retinaculum on the dorsum of the wrist, and is usually apparent as a tender swelling along the tendons. Carefully palpate the swelling and insert the needle almost parallel to the skin, aiming it into the centre of the swelling. If the needle point is in the tendon injection will be difficult. Gradually withdraw the needle, with gentle pressure on the plunger, until free, easy flow occurs. The usual dose is 25 mg hydrocortisone acetate, but volume may be a problem: inject slowly, especially after 0.5 ml.

Hand

Carpal tunnel

On the palmar surface of the hand the carpal tunnel is bridged by the flexor retinaculum, which runs between the hook of the hamate and the crest of the trapezium. These bony points are easily palpated at the level of the distal transverse skin crease. Insert the needle at right angles to the skin at this level, preferably closer to the hamate on the ulnar side, to avoid the median nerve, which is close to the trapezium, and superficial veins. The usual dose is 25 mg hydrocortisone acetate.

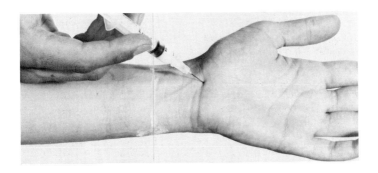

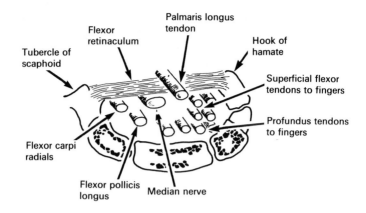

Palmar flexor tendons

Tenosynovitis of the finger flexor tendon sheaths may present as pain and difficulty on flexing the finger or as trigger finger. In the former case the tendon sheath feels thickened; in trigger finger a nodule on the tendon may be felt "popping" as the finger is flexed and extended. Carefully palpate the tendon in the palm with the fingers extended; insert the needle at the proximal skin crease of the finger, almost parallel to the course of the tendon and pointing towards the palm. Then proceed as for De Quervain's tenosynovitis.

First carpometacarpal joint of thumb

Palpate the proximal margin of the first metacarpal bone in the anatomical snuffbox: flexion of the thumb into the palm of the hand will widen the joint space. Select a site between the long extensor and long abductor muscles; locate and avoid the radial artery. Insert the needle, pointing it at the base of the little finger, to a depth of about 1 cm. The usual dose is 25 mg hydrocortisone acetate.

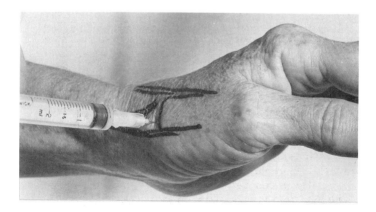

Percutaneous synovial biopsy of knee

Synovial biopsy is much simpler than open biopsy and usually yields equivalent information. Use of the Parker–

Pearson biopsy needle has been described in other joints but in practice is confined to the knee. The following instruments are required on the trolley: a Parker–Pearson needle, small scalpel blade, saline, local anaesthetic, choice of needles and syringes, sterile pack, and gloves.

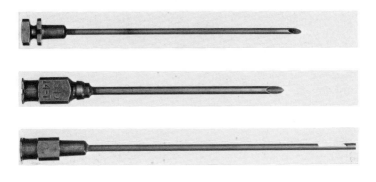

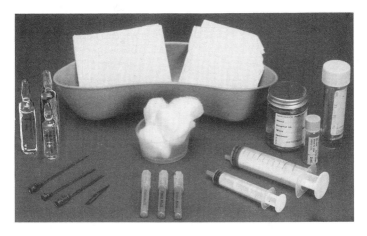

Generously infiltrate with local anaesthetic an area medial to the upper half of the patella down to the synovial membrane. If synovial fluid is required for diagnostic purposes withdraw it at this stage and replace it with 20 ml of saline. If the joint is not well distended with fluid simulate an effusion with 20 ml saline.

Incise the skin with the small scalpel needle and insert the cannula and trocar through the incision and through muscle into the joint. Reassure the patient that he may feel pressure but not pain, and infiltrate with more local anaesthetic if necessary. The cannula and trocar can usually be felt passing through the synovium, and synovial fluid will run from the cannula as the trocar is withdrawn. Angle the trocar into the suprapatellar pouch and insert the biopsy needle, so that the specimen is from the synovium under the quadriceps muscle. It is helpful to press the synovium down onto the needle with the heel of the hand and to move the cannula and needle to excise tissue rather than pull it off. The needle is then withdrawn, and synovium may be lifted out with a hypodermic needle. If the cannula is left in several specimens may be obtained.

Interpretation of results

The results of microbiological cultures and the presence or absence of micro-organisms on the gram stain film are most important. Total synovial fluid white blood cell counts and differential counts do not distinguish between, say, rheumatoid arthritis and a septic joint. A low white cell count is likely in degenerative joint disease. Raised protein levels together with low synovial glucose levels—less than 50% of plasma levels—are suggestive of infection.

Careful examination of "purulent" synovial fluid with negative microbiological results under polarised light will often reveal the crystals of uric acid or calcium pyrophosphate. Hydroxyapatite crystals may be seen on Romanovsky stains but usually can be identified only on scanning electron microscopy.

Bone marrow aspiration and trephine biopsy

S M KNOWLES

A V HOFFBRAND

Introduction

Examination of the bone marrow is essential in the diagnosis of many haematological diseases and may also be useful in the diagnosis of diseases arising outside the marrow. It provides supplementary information in many other diseases—for example, in assessing the spread of conditions in which the marrow may be secondarily affected (table I).

Aspirated marrow can be spread on slides and stained. Individual cell morphology is well retained and the exact proportion of cells of different types, the appearance of individual cells, and the presence of even a small population of abnormal cells can be recognised. The aspirated marrow is also useful for assessing iron stores and for detecting abnormalities of iron granulation of erythroblasts—for example, lack of iron granules in iron deficiency or in the anaemia of chronic disorders, or rings of iron granules in sideroblastic anaemia. Material can also be aspirated for other tests—for example, microbiological culture, cytogenetic examination, immunological markers, or gene rearrangement studies, which may characterise a case of acute leukaemia, or the deoxyuridine suppression test which can be used to distinguish between vitamin B_{12} or folate deficiency as the cause of megaloblastic anaemia (table II).

The trephine biopsy is of more value, however, for assessing the overall cellularity and architecture of the marrow—for example, whether aplastic or hyperplastic, fibrotic, or infiltrated with tumour. Individual cell morphology is more difficult to characterise. In many cases it is wise to obtain both types of specimen, for they provide complementary information.

Before embarking upon this investigation it is always preferable to discuss the case and the course of investigation with a haematologist, who can advise which samples are necessary to gain the maximum relevant information and will have access to the appropriate media required for special tests. Moreover, the spreading of satisfactory films from aspirated marrow requires experience and technical skill.

Some patients will require several bone marrow examinations in monitoring their response to treatment and it is therefore important to make the procedures as painless as

19

possible. In children it is often preferable to use a general anaesthetic or heavy sedation, but in adults local anaesthesia alone should be sufficient.

Table I—Indications for bone marrow aspiration (usually with trephine biopsy)

Diagnosis	Unexplained anaemia
	Thrombocytopenia
	Granulocytopenia
	Pancytopenia
	Certain infections (for example, leishmaniasis, tuberculosis)
	Suspected acute leukaemia
	myelodysplasia
	chronic granulocytic leukaemia
	lymphoma
	myeloproliferative disorders
	myeloma
	macroglobulinaemia
	lipoidosis
Staging	Lymphoma
	Chronic lymphocytic leukaemia
	Carcinoma
Monitoring progress	Marrow transplantation
	Acute leukaemia
	Lymphoma
	Myeloma (occasionally)

Table II—Ancillary tests which may be needed on bone marrow aspirated cells

Deoxyuridine suppression test (for B_{12} or folate deficiency)
Cytochemistry (for example, in acute leukaemia diagnosis)
Cytogenetics (for example, Philadelphia chromosome)
Immunological tests for cell surface markers (for example, acute leukaemia diagnosis)
Gene rearrangement studies (for B or T cell commitment)
Microbiological culture
Electron microscopy
Semisolid agar cultures (for example, for diagnosis of myelodysplasia)

Indications

These are listed in table I. Larger amounts of marrow (up to 400 ml) are harvested under general anaesthesia from multiple puncture sites in the pelvis when the marrow is to be used in marrow transplantation.

Contraindications

The only major complication of bone marrow aspiration or trephine is haemorrhage at the site and particularly the trephine should not be undertaken in patients with a severe coagulation defect without correcting this (see Aftercare and complications).

Equipment

- 2% plain lignocaine
- Syringes: 5 ml; 20 ml
- Needles: orange; green × 2
- Iodine (or chlorhexidine)
- Clean microscope slides and spreader
- Sterile gloves
- Sterile dressing towels
- Sterile swabs and gauze
- Media for special tests: cytogenetics; immunology; culture (for example, for tuberculosis, salmonella, other bacteria)
- Formalin container (for trephine biopsy)
- Bone marrow aspirate needle (with guard, either Salah or Klima)
- Bone marrow trephine needle (for example, Islam or Jamshidi–Swain)

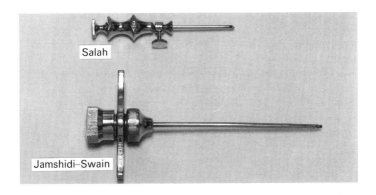

Note—Containers for peripheral blood samples should be available, since blood samples may be needed (for example, to provide autologous plasma for the dU suppression test).

Before you start

In some patients sedation may be appropriate and the best results are obtained with drugs which also have an amnesic effect (for example, midazolam 5–10 mg). For children a general anaesthetic is often needed.

Procedure

Technique for aspiration

In both adults and children the posterior iliac crest is usually used, but in infants below the age of 2 the medial aspect of the tibia, just below the tibial tubercle, may be used. For the posterior iliac crest approach the patient is placed in the right or left lateral position with the back comfortably flexed, and the medial expansion of the uppermost crest is used. The sternum is used in some subjects, particularly if obesity makes the iliac crest inaccessible.

Sedation is not usually needed except for children and apprehensive adults. A clean, no touch technique should be used, but in patients with neutropenia a mask and gloves are recommended. The patient is positioned appropriately for the site chosen and the area cleaned with chlorhexidine or iodine and surrounded with sterile towels. The bony landmarks are identified and the overlying skin and periosteum infiltrated with up to 5 ml of 2% plain lignocaine. Check that the needle is sharp, the stylet easily removable, and the guard mobile. (For iliac crest and tibial procedures the guard may be removed.) With one hand identifying the landmarks and keeping the overlying tissues taut, push the needle through the skin and subcutaneous tissues. For sternal aspiration the guard should be adjusted when the periosteum is reached, so that only a further 5 mm advancement is possible. The needle is held at right angles to the bone and with firm pressure and a clockwise–counterclockwise action pushed through the outer cortex until a sensation of decreased resistance is felt when the marrow cavity is entered. The stylet is removed, a 10 or 20 ml syringe is attached to the needle, and with sharp suction up to 0.5 ml of marrow is aspirated into the syringe for morphological examination. Any greater volume will result in increasing contamination with peripheral blood. A second volume may be aspirated into another syringe for ancillary studies.

If no marrow is aspirated the needle is rotated or the stylet replaced and the needle cautiously advanced or retracted. If marrow is still unobtainable a different site together with a clean needle should be used and possibly a trephine specimen taken.

Jamshidi–Swain trephine

The patient is positioned and prepared as for posterior crest aspiration. The skin overlying the crest is incised with a scalpel blade, or the site of entry of a previous aspiration is used. With the handle grasped in the palm of the hand and the stylet locked in position the needle is pushed through the subcutaneous tissues until it reaches the posterior crest. It is

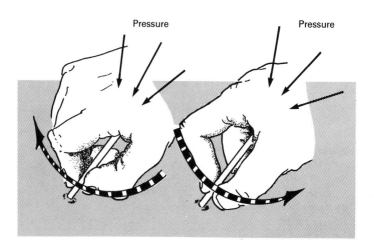

then slowly advanced with firm pressure in an alternating clockwise–counterclockwise motion in the direction of the anterior superior iliac spine until a sensation of decreased resistance is felt. The stylet is removed and the needle further advanced until 2–3 cm of marrow is obtained. The needle is then withdrawn 2–3 mm and with less pressure advanced 2–3 mm further in a different direction, which breaks the specimen at the distal cutting edge of the needle. The instrument containing the biopsy sample is then withdrawn by rotation along its axis with quick full twists. The specimen is removed from the needle by introducing the probe through the distal cutting end.

Troubleshooting

After the aspiration or trephine, firm pressure is applied to the site for three minutes or until bleeding has stopped. The site is then covered with a plaster for 24 hours.

The specimen

Aspirate

Smears must be made promptly before the specimen clots. It is a technique that requires practice, and badly made films render the aspirate uninterpretable. An accompanying technician may be needed to make the films or, if necessary, the sample may be placed into dipotassium ethylenediamine tetraacetic (K_2 EDTA) acid for a few minutes until the laboratory is reached. A paediatric tube should be used to avoid an excess of anticoagulant.

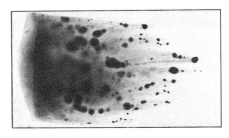

Aspiration.

When marrow films are prepared a drop of the aspirate is placed 1 cm from the end of a clean slide. Excess blood is aspirated with a Pasteur pipette or a second needle and syringe leaving marrow particles behind. Some workers concentrate all the particles on a separate slide or watch glass. By using a second smooth slide or spreader a 3–5 cm film is made from the particles in the same manner as for peripheral blood. The particles should leave a trail of cells. At least eight slides should be available for staining. Romanowsky (for example, May–Grünwald–Giemsa) and iron stains are performed routinely and cytochemical staining of other slides may be needed.

Additional material should be put in the appropriate medium with an anticoagulant for special tests—for example, cytogenetic and biochemical studies, etc—or into a microbiological culture medium.

Trephine

The specimen is placed into a histological fixative medium for decalcification and stained routinely by haematoxylin and eosin and by a silver technique for reticulin fibres. In some laboratories a plastic embedding technique is used. If the marrow aspirate has given a "dry" tap dabs are made from the trephine onto slides.

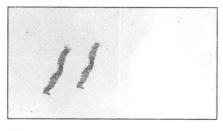

Trephine biopsy.

Aftercare and complications

In severe coagulation disorders (for example, haemophilia, severe disseminated intravascular coagulation) the procedure should be undertaken only when the defect has been corrected by appropriate plasma fraction replacements. A trephine biopsy in such conditions might give rise to prolonged haemorrhage. Thrombocytopenia alone does not usually present a major problem.

Failure to use the guard when performing sternal aspiration could give rise to complete penetration of the bone with a resultant fatal haemorrhage, pericardial tamponade, mediastinitis, or pneumomediastinum. Local sepsis is extremely rare except in patients with severe neutropenia, for whom stringent sterile precautions should be taken.

After the procedure a plaster is applied, and firm pressure over the site for a few minutes is recommended (for longer if the patient has a haemostatic defect).

Interpretation of results

The marrow aspirate films may be ready for examination after staining within 2–4 hours of obtaining the specimen. The marrow must be looked at microscopically by an experienced haematologist to assess the cellularity, proportion of various cell types, the appearance of the individual cells, and presence of any abnormal cells. The iron stain may be examined later. A decision on further stains on the unfixed blood films or further specialised tests to be performed on the sample of the aspirated marrow taken into anticoagulant or special media may be taken after an initial examination of the Romanowsky stained films.

The trephine biopsy will usually be processed in the department of histopathology and is available for sectioning and staining after decalcification, which may take several days. The stained sections are examined microscopically by the histopathologist, a haematologist, or both.

Removal of drains and sutures

N M KORUTH

PETER F JONES

Reasons for insertion

Although drains and sutures are inserted at the end of an operation, when the important parts of the procedure seem to be over, they play an important and at times vital part in the recovery of the patient. It is wise to have a rule that the surgeon who inserted a drain or sutures is the person who decides on the removal.

Drains provide a mechanical means of removing material that would otherwise be harmful to the patient, and this may be pus, air, blood, urine, or alimentary secretions. There are three main reasons for inserting drains—namely, to remove air and blood that will delay healing and recovery, to drain abscesses, and to provide a safe and convenient route for secretions to leave the body—and these differing reasons will dictate the way in which the drains are managed.

Removal of air and blood

Although in many operations—for instance, inguinal hernia repair—there is no need to insert any drain, in many clean, planned operations considerable areas are opened up. After total mastectomy air is trapped under the skin flaps and

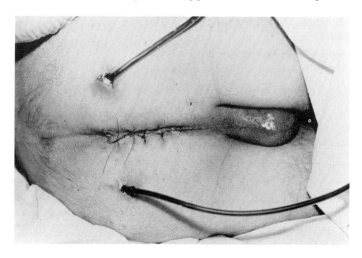

blood and serum will, however good the haemostasis, drain from the chest wall and prevent the skin flaps from adhering if drainage is not provided. A haematoma can be dangerous after thyroidectomy and delay healing after excision of the rectum. In all these circumstances efficient drainage is important, but it is equally important that the drain track should provide no entry for bacteria, so a secure system of closed drainage is essential. Most surgeons now use a suction type of drain, in which a fine tube with multiple side holes is inserted through a stab wound and attached through closed tubing to a suction bottle: this has proved effective and bacteriologically safe.

The drains are removed when they cease to be useful—usually 24–48 hours after thyroidectomy. After an extensive operation like mastectomy it is important to measure the volume of fluid drained each day, and it is often five to six days before this has dwindled sufficiently to permit removal. These drains are secured by a suture, and on removal this stitch is cut and the drain swiftly withdrawn so that air does not re-enter the wound through the side holes in the tubing.

Intrapleural drains require special care because disconnection will result in pneumothorax. All these drains are attached to underwater seal bottles, and, if suction is not being applied to the open end of the bottle, there should be a respiratory swing in the level of fluid in the tubing.

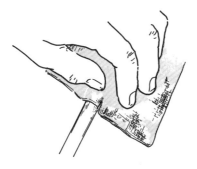

Management of these drains is always under the control of the surgeon. When the drain is ready for removal the suture securing it to the skin is cut, a pad made of a thick square of tulle gras surmounted by several layers of gauze is pressed firmly over wound and drain, and the drain is swiftly withdrawn; the pad is strapped firmly over the drain hole. In this way entry of air into the pleura during removal should be avoided.

Drainage of abscesses and secretions

Sometimes drains have to remain in position for a long time. After drainage of a subphrenic abscess or an empyema a large cavity is left, which will contract and heal only slowly; the tube must not be removed until the cavity is obliterated. This process is assessed by serial contrast radiology, via the drainage tube, every seven to 10 days.

27

Drains inserted to remove secretions are usually placed in the abdomen. After operations such as cholecystectomy and ureterolithotomy the surgeon hopes that there will be no drainage of bile or urine but cannot be certain of this. Accumulation of bile or urine in the body can cause serious complications, so a suction or tube drain is placed beside the operation site and attached to a sterile transparent plastic bag. If no appreciable drainage is seen in the bag after 48–72 hours these drains may safely be removed.

When urine is being deliberately diverted through a tube— for example, after suprapubic cystostomy or nephrostomy— the timing of removal depends on the reason for drainage and is decided solely by the operator.

After gastrectomy or intestinal resection and anastomosis there is a period of five to seven days during which the anastomosis is healing but still depends on the integrity of the sutures, so it is essential for the drainage tube beside the anastomosis to remain until this period is over and leakage from the suture line is unlikely. There is always a tendency for fibrinous adhesions to occlude an intraperitoneal drain, so it is wise to shorten such drains after four or five days; this often disturbs adhesions and allows a sealed off collection of fluid to drain. It is essential to fix the shortened drain securely (use 0·5 in zinc oxide adhesive tape) so that it cannot be accidentally pulled out.

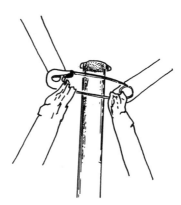

The advantages of using a soft tube instead of corrugated rubber are that the fluid passing along it can be collected, measured, and analysed, and the secretion does not contaminate the abdominal wall. This can be extremely important if, for instance, a fistula should form in the pancreas or small intestine. Modern disposable drainage bags easily permit collection and measurement and keep the drainage system closed, preventing reflux of air and bacteria along the tubing.

One of the serious aspects of duodenal and pancreatic fistulae is that the enzymes are proteolytic and can cause serious digestion of wounds. With the development of intravenous feeding it is possible to wait while fistulae gradually contract and heal, during which time it is sometimes helpful to use a sump drain. This allows secretions to be aspirated near to their point of origin, which protects the tissues from digestion and keeps the patient comfortable.

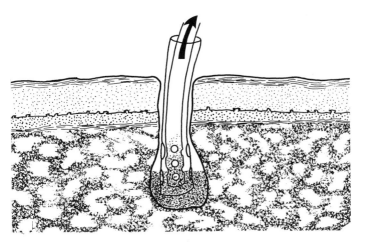

Insertion of T tube

After exploration of the common bile duct a T tube of latex rubber is usually inserted to permit direct drainage of the infected and distended duct. The external end of the tube is placed into a sterile plastic bag (sealed drainage) hanging beside the bed, and the volume of bile drained is recorded every 24 hours: occasionally this volume is high and constitutes an important source of water and electrolyte loss. After eight to 10 days' drainage cholangiography is usually performed to ensure that there is free drainage into the duodenum and no sign of a residual stone. The T tube is withdrawn by steady traction 24 hours later.

Accidental removal

Drains are only inserted for specific important reasons, so they must be secured by a method which prevents accidental removal. This usually means that a strong suture is passed deeply through skin adjacent to the point of emergence of the drain, and it is wound several times round the drain, and tied securely. This should be proof against an accidental tug during bedmaking, or traction by a disorientated patient.

If, nevertheless, premature removal of a drain occurs then the surgeon must be informed. It is rarely possible to replace a drain without a further operation. Consequently, if the drain is a precautionary one placed in a healing wound—for example, after mastectomy—or beside openings in the urinary or alimentary tracts it is usual to await events. It is quite likely that no harmful collection will occur, but special vigilance is needed. The premature removal of a T tube draining the common bile duct may not result in any untoward effects, but if it is followed by signs of developing peritonitis an urgent laparotomy is mandatory.

The early removal of a tube draining an abscess cavity—for example, a subphrenic abscess—will generally require reinsertion of the tube: this may be possible under x ray control.

Burst abdomen

Dehiscence of an abdominal incision carries a mortality of 10–20%. The elderly, and patients with malignant disease or jaundice or an infected incision, are particularly at risk. So are those with postoperative respiratory infections or intestinal ileus. With the abandonment of catgut and the use of modern methods of incisional closure the incidence of dehiscence has fallen to less than 1%. This reduction is due to the use of non-absorbable (or slowly absorbed) sutures, some form of mass closure of the incision, secure knotting, and prevention of wound infection.

Warning of wound disruption, which tends to occur around the seventh postoperative day, is given by leakage of serosanguineous fluid from the wound edges—occasionally a loop of intestine can be seen protruding. If skin sutures are removed the muscle layers are seen to have parted, and abdominal viscera are visible. The surgeon should be immediately informed. Generally, immediate steps are taken to resuture the wound under general anaesthesia, using multiple deep all layer sutures of nylon or polypropylene.

Special attention must be given to postoperative analgesia and chest physiotherapy. Intravenous fluids are continued until gastrointestinal activity returns: parenteral nutrition may have an important role if this is delayed.

Removal of skin sutures

Suture marks—the imprinted scar of the pressure of suture material on the skin surface—are determined by the time for which a suture is left in place, its tension, and its position. The aim must be to remove sutures as soon as their purpose is achieved, and on the face and neck scars heal quickly, so that sutures can usually be removed in 24–72 hours. These sutures are small and fine, and it is essential when removing them to have the patient lying comfortably, to work in a good light, and to have a sharp pair of scissors with fine points and fine, non-toothed dissecting forceps. Always divide the suture close to the skin below the knot and then gently pull the

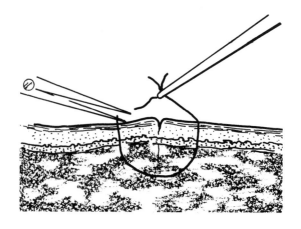

suture out towards the side on which it was divided, using the points of the scissors to give counter pressure on the wound.

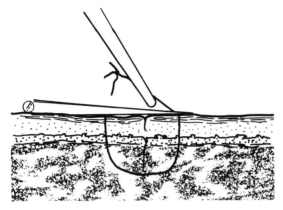

Incisions that are made in the line of skin creases heal quickly, and sutures in, for example, an inguinal hernia wound can usually be removed in six or seven days. Vertical abdominal wounds heal more slowly and sutures are removed in seven to 10 days; and sutures in the skin of the back and calf need to remain for 10–12 days. If deep nylon retention sutures are placed in an abdominal wound the surgeon will probably keep them in position for 12–14 days.

Skin biopsy

ALLAN S HIGHET

ROBERT H CHAMPION

Indications

Skin histology is not a substitute for clinical assessment but is complementary to it.

Histology is especially valuable in diagnosing tumours; it is always required if malignancy is suspected but is not essential if a benign diagnosis is clinically undoubted—for example, typical seborrhoeic keratosis. Histology and immunohistology (usually immunofluorescence) are indicated in chronic bullous disease such as pemphigus, pemphigoid, and dermatitis herpetiformis. Leucocyte markers are of some value in the diagnosis of suspected lymphomas.

In the diagnosis of inflammatory skin diseases biopsy will usually be limited to unusual or atypical conditions. With the possible exception of tumours removed by, for example, general practitioners or surgeons, a dermatological opinion should normally be obtained before a skin biopsy.

Contraindications

Common complicatons, including the inevitability of scarring, must be weighed against the likely benefit; thus one will usually have a higher threshold for performing a biopsy on eruptions confined to the face.

Biopsy will usually be avoided or postponed in the presence of cutaneous infection. Rare conditions that may delay healing will militate against biopsy, including severe disorders of collagen formation or of haemostasis. Most patients on anticoagulants can have skin biopsies performed without any problems. If patients are suspected of carrying the virus of the acquired immune deficiency syndrome even minor surgical procedures should usually be performed in special accommodation and with special precautions now specified by many hospitals.

Equipment

For the standard elliptical excision biopsy the following are required:
- Scalpel
- Fine toothed forceps
- Needle holder

- Scissors
- Eyeless needle with suture
- Sterile drapes
- Towel clips
- Artery forceps
- Gauze swabs
- Surgical gloves
- Local anaesthetic
- Syringe
- Needles
- Antiseptic
- Specimen jar

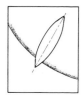

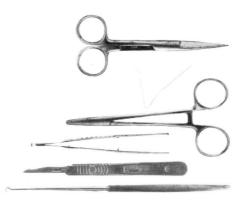

Some prefer to handle the specimen with a skin hook, but forceps trauma is minimised if the specimen is handled only at the ends.

Alcohol based antiseptics—for example, chlorhexidine 0·5% in 70% ethanol—are generally the most effective but should be avoided if diathermy or cautery is intended before evaporation of the alcohol can be ensured—in hairy areas, for instance.

Before you start

The implications of the procedure and the likely consequences (for example, scarring) should be discussed with the patient beforehand.

The laboratory may need prior warning if the specimen has to be processed promptly—for example, unfixed tissue for immunofluorescence or leucocyte markers.

Aseptic precautions should be similar to those for any other surgical procedure.

A local anaesthetic is injected just under the skin. Superficial blebs resulting from injecting fluid into the skin itself must be avoided at the biopsy site. Occasionally it is necessary to avoid the biopsy site itself and to inject the anaesthetic in a ring around it—for example, to preserve mast cells.

Vasoconstrictors such as adrenaline and felypressin reduce bleeding but must not be used in fingers, toes, ears, or penis because intense vasospasm may result in tissue necrosis.

Basic techniques

Elliptical excision biopsy

The ellipse should normally measure about 12 × 4 mm, but smaller specimens may be adequate if required for cosmetic or other reasons. The ends of the ellipse should be pointed to aid closure of the wound. When two specimens are needed from the same site—for example, one for routine histological examination and one for immunofluorescence— two longitudinal halves of the excised ellipse are convenient. It is easier to make the central incision first.

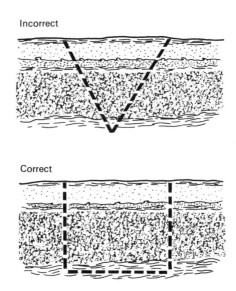

Incorrect

Correct

Incisions should always be made vertical to the skin surface. Incisions slanted inwards result in an unsatisfactory, wedge shaped specimen and imperfect apposition of the wound edges. The full thickness of skin is incised. The elliptical island of skin, now attached only by the subcutaneous tissue, is lifted by one corner, ideally with a skin hook or needle, and separated, by scalpel or scissors, from the deep tissue to leave attached to the underside of the dermis a thin layer of subcutaneous fat. If pathological changes in the fat are suspected a deeper specimen will be necessary.

Interrupted non-absorbable sutures (for example, silk) are usually used. Equal bites are made on each side of the wound, the needle piercing the skin 2–3 mm from the cut edge.

Punch biopsy

The punch is a metal cylinder with a sharp cutting edge at one end. A 3 or 4 mm diameter instrument is preferred for most work, but smaller and larger sizes are available. The punch is pushed with a downward and twisting movement (imparted either by hand or by motor) into the skin, then removed. The specimen is lifted and separated by scissors from the underlying tissue. The wound may be left unsutured or the base cauterised for haemostasis, but inserting one or two stitches gives a better result. Scarring is further minimised by using the punch while traction is applied outwards across the wrinkle lines; when the traction is released the open wound takes up an oval shape.

This method has the advantage of saving time, but most pathologists prefer the elliptical excision method.

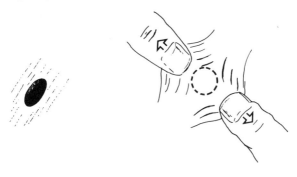

Curettage

Curettage with a sharp edged spoon curette followed by cautery may be used to remove certain skin lesions including warts, basal cell carcinomas, seborrhoeic keratoses, and actinic keratoses. Though generally satisfactory for histological examination, curetted specimens are usually incomplete or fragmented (although with care this may be minimised). Curettage, therefore, is mainly a therapeutic procedure and is only indirectly a biopsy technique.

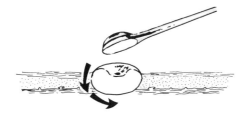

Epidermal (shave) biopsy

Superficial lesions (for example, cellular naevi and largely epidermal disorders) may be shaved off by horizontal cutting with a scalpel, the skin being raised if necessary by gentle pinching. The defect may be cauterised for haemostasis.

Needle biopsy

Biopsy needles, like those used for liver biopsy, have been used but are not generally satisfactory.

Choice of lesion

In general, a representative lesion at the height of its intensity, unmodified by trauma or treatment, will best show the histological features. The major exceptions are blisters (and pustules), which should be as new as possible and preferably less than a day old when the specimen is taken. An older blister may show confusing changes owing to regeneration, excoriation, or infection.

When the edge of the lesion is well demarcated it is usually best to take the specimen from the edge to include a small portion of normal skin. The edge is often the most active part of the lesion, and the normal skin serves as a built-in control. Sutures often hold better on normal skin. In blistering eruptions, however, perilesional skin is the best site for immunofluorescence and should form the greater proportion of the specimen. When the lesions are poorly demarcated a site of maximum activity should be sought.

Sometimes it may be necessary to take multiple specimens to assess the evolution or varied morphology of lesions.

Orientation of incision

The long axis of the wound should follow the natural wrinkle lines of the skin.

Choice of body site

Some scarring is inevitable, and the site should be chosen to minimise cosmetic disability. With keloids individual predisposition is the main factor, but the chin, midline of the chest, shoulders, and upper outer arms are areas in which the risk of keloid formation is greatest.

Sites subject to much movement, friction, or pressure are best avoided.

Healing on the lower legs is often slow but may be improved by rest and elevation or supportive bandaging.

Skin tumours

Suspected malignant melanoma

Clinical diagnosis of malignant melanoma is notoriously inaccurate. A lesion that is strongly suspected of being a melanoma should be widely excised and may often require grafting. When a lesion might only possibly be a melanoma it is better not to inflict such an operation on the patient. The lesion should be completely excised with a minimum margin of 1–2 mm. Further surgery would of course be required should the lesion prove to be a melanoma.

Other malignant tumours

When surgical excision would be the treatment of choice for a suspected malignant tumour direct referral to the surgeon is preferable to a preliminary biopsy.

Keratoacanthoma

This is a benign, spontaneously regressing tumour. It may be histologically confused with squamous carcinoma unless the specimen clearly shows its typical architecture. The specimen should include a segment of the shoulder of the lesion extending into the central crater, along with adjacent normal skin and subcutaneous fat. If the clinical diagnosis of keratoacanthoma can confidently be made curettage, while failing to meet all the above criteria, may be regarded as satisfactory.

The specimen

A small specimen may curl. This may be prevented by laying it flat, underside down—that is, epidermis upwards—on a small piece of blotting paper and placing the whole in the fixative. The standard fixative is formol saline.

For examination by immunofluorescence the specimen is preserved by freezing, without chemical fixative. Several techniques are used. In one a 7% gelatin solution (liquefied if necessary by warming) is poured into a small plastic capsule. The specimen is immersed directly in the gelatin and the (labelled) capsule closed and dropped into a flask containing liquid nitrogen. The specimen must remain frozen during transport to the laboratory.

If a specimen has to be cultured for micro-organisms it should not be fixed at all or allowed to dry out. For other special investigations—for example, electron microscopy—the laboratory should be consulted.

The accompanying form must contain adequate identification and a clinical summary including the suspected or differential diagnosis. A sketch of the biopsy area may be helpful. Specimens must, of course, be correctly labelled.

Aftercare and complications

Sutures should be removed after four or five days for the face, 10 days for the leg, and seven days for most other sites.

An occlusive dressing kept in place for several days may enhance bacterial growth. The initial dressing should be discarded after a day. If continued cover is desired the dressing should be changed daily. It is not necessary to prohibit washing if the wound is treated gently.

Haemorrhage

Small arteries may be cut, resulting in pulsatile bleeding. This will usually subside spontaneously or respond to direct pressure or wound closure. Occasionally the vessel may have to be clamped and a ligature of absorbable catgut applied.

Scalp incisions may bleed profusely.

Sepsis

Factors predisposing to infection include careless technique and occlusive dressings. Sepsis may require early removal of one or more sutures, and any infection with cellulitis, lymphangitis, or lymphadenitis or threatening to cause breakdown of the wound should be treated with a systemic antibiotic.

Incomplete healing

Gaping wounds seldom benefit from direct resuturing but if the gap is large the edges should be excised and the wound reclosed.

Keloids

The risk of keloid formation may be reduced by attention to the details enumerated above.

Setting up a drip

BARBARA A BANNISTER

Indications

Many hospital inpatients, and some outpatients, have intravenous cannulae at some stage of their management. Indications for the use of cannulae fall into three main groups:
(1) To introduce or replace fluids in the circulation—for example, blood, blood products, colloids, or electrolyte solutions.
(2) To provide a route for administering intravenous medication or nutrition.
(3) To permit monitoring of central venous pressures: in this case a long, flexible catheter is used to reach along a peripheral vein into the superior vena cava.

Precautions

No absolute contraindications exist, but particular care is needed in some circumstances:
(1) If heart failure is present or incipient an extra circulating fluid load may result in severe pulmonary oedema. If a blood transfusion or intravenous infusion is essential this problem may be alleviated by giving diuretics simultaneously.
(2) In renal failure it is important that the fluid and electrolyte loads, as well as the amount of drugs given, do not exceed the excretory capabilities of the kidneys.
(3) If small veins with inadequate blood flow are cannulated toxic or irritant substances may pool at the infusion site, causing inflammation or necrosis.
(4) In patients with impaired immune responses or damaged heart valves a drip site is an important portal for the entry of potentially fatal infection. Strict attention to asepsis and restriction of the time for which the cannula is in situ are necessary. If prolonged use of a long catheter is expected the outer end should be drawn through a skin "tunnel," so that the site of the skin puncture is several centimetres from the vein—for example, Broviac or Hickman catheters. The stab wounds are closed with a stitch when the catheter is in position, and the giving set connection is outside the tunnel, strapped to the chest wall. Superficial infection of the entry site is then unlikely to progress rapidly to the cannulated vein.

38

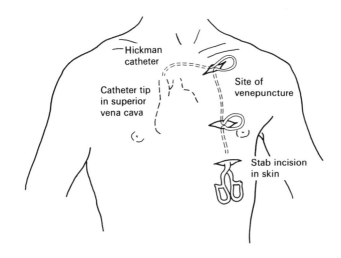

Equipment

Sterile fluid and giving set

The fluid or blood is usually presented in a collapsible plastic bag. If the fluid is in a rigid bottle an air inlet tube will be required to prevent the formation of a vacuum when fluid flows out of the bottle into the giving set.

To prepare the giving set first remove the sterile cover from the bag or bottle outlet. Then close the adjustable valve of the giving set, remove the sterile cover from the bag connector, and push the connector firmly into the bag or bottle outlet. This should be done with the neck of the bag pointing upwards, and the bag connector downwards, so that no fluid enters the giving set. The fingers should not touch the bag outlet port or the connector during this manoeuvre or skin bacteria from the operator might be introduced into the connection.

The bag should now be inverted to hang on the drip stand, and the drip chamber of the giving set squeezed to obtain a fluid level. (If an air inlet is required for a rigid bottle it should be inserted at this stage.) Now raise the Luer-Lok connector, with its sterile cover, above the fluid level in the drip chamber and open the adjustable valve. The fluid will fill the plastic tubing up to the level in the drip chamber. By slowly lowering the Luer-Lok connector, the tubing can be filled exactly with minimal bubble formation. The adjustable valve is then closed. Any small bubbles will float to the fluid surfaces if the tube is held vertical and tapped sharply. The set is now ready for use.

Cannulae

These are made of plastic material, and may be teflon coated to improve the flow characteristics of fluid through them and discourage thrombus formation. For small veins, or when a short cannula is required, the winged type of metal cannula is convenient. It is best to use a cannula without side ports or three way tap connections, as these features cause stagnant areas where thrombus or organisms may be deposited.

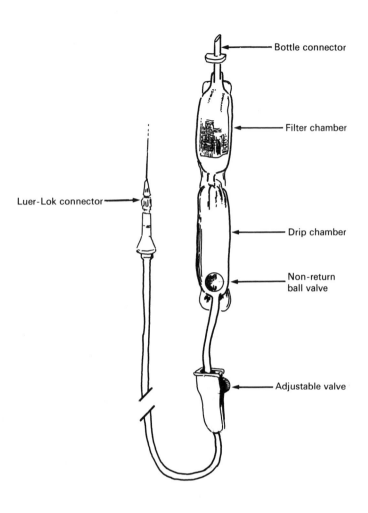

Bottle connector

Filter chamber

Luer-Lok connector

Drip chamber

Non-return
ball valve

Adjustable valve

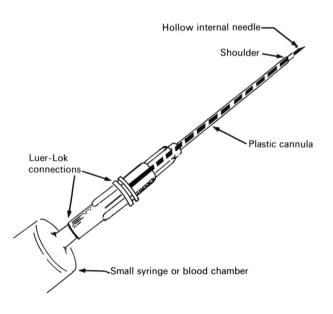

Hollow internal needle

Shoulder

Plastic cannula

Luer-Lok
connections

Small syringe or blood chamber

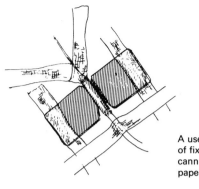

A useful method
of fixing a winged
cannula with thin
paper strapping

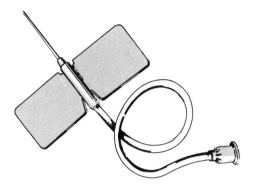

Long catheters are made of plastic or silicon materials and contain radio-opaque markers so that their position in the veins can be checked by radiographs. It is not advisable to insert plastic intravenous catheters through metal needles, as catheters can quite easily be severed by the sharp needle tip during manipulation. A catheter embolism may result, requiring risky and complicated intervention for its removal.

Other equipment
- Alcohol impregnated swabs for skin cleansing
- Cotton wool balls for applying local pressure
- Gauze pads, paper tape, and crepe bandage
- "Sharps bin," or a tray for carrying "sharps" away for disposal.

Choice of vein

The most convenient site for peripheral cannulae is the left forearm (or the right in a left handed patient). This permits comfortable mobility of the left arm and leaves the right free for writing, washing, etc. Veins at the elbow should be avoided if possible, as the cannula is difficult to fix firmly, and uncomfortable immobilisation of the joint is required. The dorsum of the hand is a convenient site, and the winged type of cannula is most easily inserted and fixed here, particularly in children. Veins near the ankle may also be used; in the restless patient the leg is often easier to immobilise and dress than the arm. An experienced operator may cannulate the jugular, subclavian, or saphenous vein, or a scalp vein in an infant. The cephalic vein can be difficult to cannulate with a long catheter as it is sharply angled at the shoulder; the basilic vein is much easier.

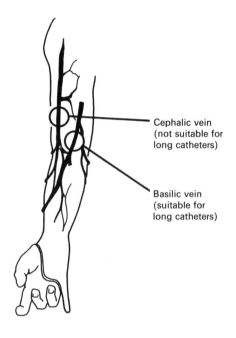

Cephalic vein
(not suitable for
long catheters)

Basilic vein
(suitable for
long catheters)

Veins are much easier to cannulate at a site where they penetrate fascia, or at a confluence, as they are then fixed and cannot roll away from the needle point.

Venepuncture

The procedure is explained to the patient; veins are much easier to identify if the patient is warm and comfortable. Clothing is removed from the limb and a tourniquet applied to occlude venous return. A suitable superficial vein is selected and a generous area around the chosen site should be well cleaned with an alcohol swab or alcoholic solution. When long catheters are to be used sterile drapes and gloves make it easier to perform a "sterile" procedure. While the alcohol dries a cannula is selected which will lie comfortably in the vein without completely filling it.

The needle and cannula should first be inserted through the skin beyond the shoulder of the plastic part. The metal needle is allowed to touch the vein, with the flat side of the bevel pointing to the skin surface. Downwards oblique pressure will then cause the needle to enter the vein, and pressure is continued to guide the plastic shoulder of the cannula into the vein lumen. Blood will enter the chamber, or can be drawn into the syringe. The tourniquet is then released and the metal needle is withdrawn from the cannula, while leakage of blood is prevented by pressing a cotton wool ball on the vein over the tip of the cannula. The needle is immediately dropped into the "sharps bin" or onto a tray for later removal. The giving set is connected and the adjustable valve is opened to allow slow flow of fluid into the vein.

Fixing and dressing

The cannula must be fixed securely, as movement may damage it, leading to leakage and the entry of micro-organisms. A crepe bandage may be applied overall and will help to warm the fluid as it flows towards the vein. Splints should be avoided if possible, as immobilisation reduces blood flow, encouraging stasis and thrombosis.

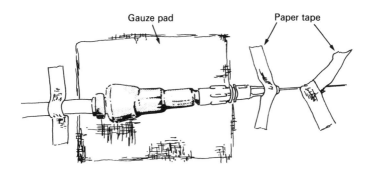

Gauze pad   Paper tape

Infection control

This has two purposes:
(1) To protect the operator from exposure to the patient's blood, which may be infectious.
(2) To protect the patient from the entry of pathogens into the venepuncture site or the vascular system.
Several simple procedures contribute greatly to the safety and sterility of the procedure:
(1) Careful preparation is important. An orderly tray or trolley with all the necessary equipment will save fluster and maintain hygiene.
(2) The operator's hands should be washed immediately before cleaning the venepuncture site, and again at the end of the procedure, before attending to the next patient.
(3) The tourniquet should always be released before removing the needle or cannula. This prevents leakage of blood due to back pressure in the vein. Cotton wool balls will absorb tiny leakages of blood and should therefore always be used when applying pressure to venepuncture sites.
(4) Inoculation accidents readily occur if the operator attempts to "resheath" the used needle in its cover or

43

package. It is better to discard the needle by dropping it directly into a "sharps bin" or rigid tray. It is dangerous to leave needles among dressings and packing where they might be hidden and later cause injury during cleaning up.

(5) Bloodstained dressings should also be discarded immediately into suitable disposal bags.

(6) The venepuncture site should be inspected daily. All short cannulae should be resited at two or three day intervals so that micro-organisms do not have time to become established in the tissues or vein. Giving sets should be changed every one or two days, and immediately after blood transfusion as organic matter is trapped in the filter chamber and may harbour micro-organisms. Adding 500 units of heparin to each 500 ml of fluid infused discourages thrombus formation and associated sepsis.

Problems

No veins visible or palpable

An experienced operator may perform "blind" cannulation of the jugular or subclavian vein. Alternatively, a "cut down" procedure may be employed. A small incision is made at the elbow or ankle and, with a tourniquet on the limb, a vein is displayed by blunt dissection of subcutaneous tissue and is cannulated under direct vision.

Failure to penetrate the vein

This is common when elderly patients have fibrous or calcified veins. Remove the tourniquet and apply pressure to the venepuncture site during and after removal of the cannula in case the vein is leaking. Try again at another site with a smaller cannula. If repeatedly unsuccessful ask a more experienced colleague for help; provided that all possible sites have not been spoiled a chance to demonstrate skill at venepunctures is often welcomed. Anaesthetists perform many venepunctures and will often succeed where others have failed.

Failure of fluid to flow

Check that the tourniquet has been removed, that the adjustable valve is open, and that an air inlet has been used if appropriate. The appearance of a bleb of subcutaneous fluid shows that the cannula is not in the vein lumen and the drip should be resited. Finally, the cannula may be flushed with fluid, in case it is blocked by thrombus.

Appearance of inflammation

The cannula must be removed immediately, as local infection will not clear or respond to treatment while foreign material is present in the tissues. Persisting infection may lead to bacteraemia and is also a source of cross infection for other patients. An unexplained fever in a patient with a drip is often due to inflammation at the venepuncture site. Always wash the hands between removing the infected cannula and performing a new venepuncture procedure.

Careful attention to the siting, dressing, and management of a drip can make the difference between wellbeing and misery for the patient and is very rewarding for the little time it takes.

Putting up a drip and taking blood in young children

CHARLES NOBLE-JAMIESON
ANDREW WHITELAW

Putting up a drip

Intravenous infusions are often needed in young children and infants for rehydration, drug treatment, inability to tolerate feeding, and surgery. Modern plastic intravenous cannulae are small enough for use on limb or scalp veins in even the tiniest preterm infants and have the advantage that they do not cut out of the vein even when there is some movement. The cheaper butterfly needle may still be needed for scalp vein infusions, although these should be avoided where possible as parents are often distressed at seeing hair shaved off.

Equipment

Assemble the materials for the drip in advance, in a room with a good light. The cannula used (22 or 24 G) should have short wings at the hub. You will need a strip of ½ inch adhesive tape, a splint to secure the drip, and a 1 ml syringe

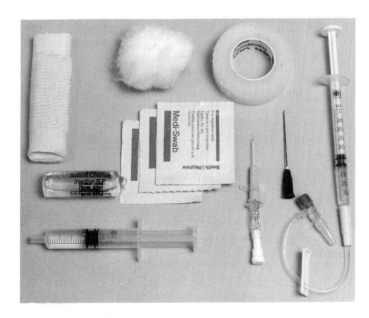

filled with 0·9% saline to flush. A further syringe filled with heparinised saline and attached to a T connector is useful to keep the cannula patent while the giving set is prepared.

Preparation of the child

A young child should be held by a parent where possible. Select a suitable vein on the hand, arm, or foot. The child should be held sideways on the mother's lap with one arm behind her back. The mother will be responsible for holding the child's trunk and, if she wishes, screening the child's view with her free hand. A nurse will hold the drip hand or foot braced against the mother's knee. Explain to the child that you are going to "make a scratch in his hand which will hurt for a moment, and then put a big bandage on it." A small baby may be swaddled tightly in a sheet, leaving the chosen limb free, and held by the nurse. Scalp veins in the parietal or temporal region may be chosen, in which case some of the hair will need to be shaved using a disposable razor.

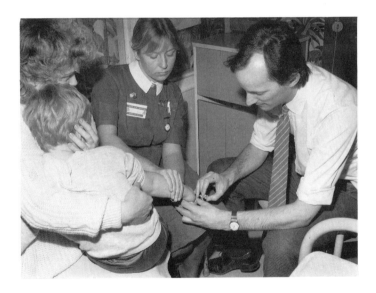

Insertion of the cannula

Ideal veins for cannulation are those that are easily immobilised—for example, the median cubital vein, which is fixed in fascia, or a vein on the hand with a Y junction, which prevents the vein from moving away during insertion of the needle. Ensure that the vein is well filled with blood, if necessary by a peristaltic pumping action from above. The assistant must not squeeze so hard as to cut off the arterial supply. Swab the skin well with alcohol and allow to dry. Pierce the skin about 5 mm from the point at which the vein will be entered, using a separate needle, as the fine plastic cannula is easily damaged. Pass the cannula on its needle through the same hole in the skin and lift the tip of the needle so that it is moving superficially in the subcutaneous layer. Aim to enter the vein from above, preferably in the angle of the Y junction. Once the needle is in the lumen and blood is seen flashing back from the needle hub, lift up the bevel of the needle and advance it until the cannula itself is in the lumen of the vein. Most cannulae now have a raised shoulder at the hub which can be pressed gently with the forefinger to hold the cannula stationary in the lumen of the vein while the needle is withdrawn. If this process has been successfully accomplished blood will be seen flushing back up the cannula as the needle is withdrawn. If no blood flushes back it is likely that the vein has been transfixed and that the cannula tip is below the vein. Remove the needle completely and pull back the cannula slowly until blood flushes back. Lay the cannula hub as flat as possible on the skin and advance the cannula into the lumen of the vein.

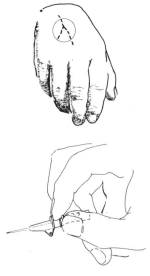

When the cannula is in the lumen attach the 1 ml syringe and inject a little saline. Keep flushing saline slowly into the vein and gently push the cannula through the skin up to the hub.

Securing the cannula

Clean away any spilt blood from the skin and cannula using a spirit swab and allow to dry. Place a strip of tape under the wings of the cannula adhesive side up and fold the tape over the wings and stick it parallel to the line of the cannula. Put a further strip of tape over the hub of the cannula. Replace the 1 ml syringe with the T connector. Strap the hand or arm gently to the splint. Try to avoid putting tape circumferentially around the arm proximal to the catheter tip as this will impede flow from the cannula and encourage thrombophlebitis. Insert some cotton wool behind the hub of the cannula and strap gently. Tape the T connector firmly to the splint.

If potentially irritant fluids containing calcium salts, amino acids, or some drugs are infused serious necrosis of the skin can follow extravasation. An intravenous site should be inspected every hour without removing any adhesive by the nurse looking after the infant. Increasing swelling or redness should be investigated and the infusion should be stopped if extravasation is suspected.

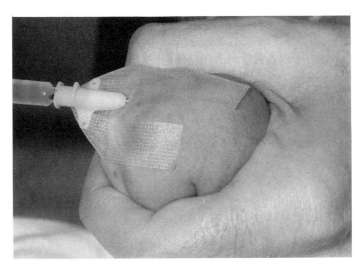

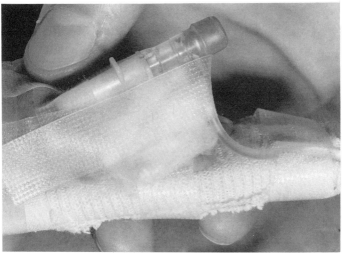

Scalp vein infusion with butterfly needle

Explain to the mother that the needle is not going inside the skull, the needle is painless after insertion, and the hair will grow back. Shave the hair on the temporoparietal area on one side. Palpate the vessel and check the direction of blood flow to ensure that a vein and not an artery will be infused. Avoid the forehead as extravasation of irritant solutions may leave a scar. Immobilise all but the smallest infants by wrapping in a sheet.

Prepare the butterfly needle (short 25 or 23 G) by filling it with 0·9% saline. Cut strips of narrow adhesive and gauze impregnated with plaster of Paris. Make a tourniquet with an elastic band around the head or a finger proximal to the site of insertion. Select a Y junction or straight vein and insert the needle 0·5 cm away from the planned point of entry as this will help to stabilise the needle. Insert the needle into the vein from above and see that blood will flow back along the tubing. Inject some saline and check for subcutaneous swelling. Tape down the wings of the needle and pack a little cotton wool or plaster of Paris behind the needle to keep the butterfly needle at the optimum angle for infusion. Plaster of Paris may be spread over the wings giving effective immobilisation. The needle should remain visible to detect extravasion. A plastic cup with two sections cut out gives protection while providing visibility.

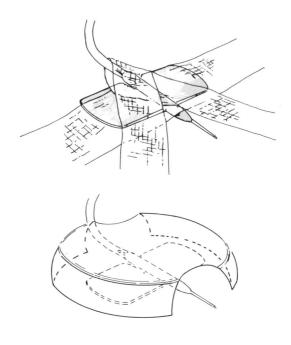

Emergency vascular access

Even a skilled paediatrician may find it difficult to site a drip in a moribund, hypovolaemic infant. Remember that some emergency drugs such as 1:10000 adrenaline, atropine, and naloxone can be given via an endotracheal tube in an emergency. Internal jugular puncture or subclavian puncture should only be attempted by those skilled in their use. The external jugular vein or scalp veins may prove accessible if the child is held in a head down position. The bone marrow provides a convenient route for the administration of drugs, fluid, and blood: a wide bore butterfly needle should be inserted into the bone marrow of the tibia 1–3 cm below the tibial tuberosity after careful skin preparation. Strong hypertonic solutions such as 50% dextrose or 10% calcium gluconate should of course be avoided, but otherwise this route to the circulation is suitable for a wide range of dextrose–electrolyte solutions, plasma, blood, and drugs.[1]

Taking blood

Venipuncture

Blood samples may readily be obtained using a 23 G butterfly needle and syringe, adopting the above technique. Use the smallest possible syringe so you can aspirate very gently, otherwise the vein will collapse. If the blood is required for culture sterilise the skin with povidine–iodine solution and allow to dry.

Blood may be obtained from small babies by allowing blood to drip directly from the needle into the sampling bottles. Use a wide bore needle (for example, 21 G) and break off the hub before inserting the needle into the vein. If the baby's hand is held in the operator's palm with the fingers flexed blood can be "pumped" into the baby's hand by a peristaltic action. This technique is not suitable for obtaining blood for culture.

Capillary blood sampling

In babies under 6 months the heel is the ideal site for capillary blood sampling, but in older infants the thumb is better. The heel must be warm: if it is cold dip the foot into hand warm water (40°C) for five minutes and then dry it thoroughly. Hold the foot by encircling the ball of the heel with your thumb and forefinger. Select a site on the side of the heel, wipe it with isopropyl alcohol, and allow it to dry. Do no use the ball or back of the heel because a painful ulcer may form. Apply a thin layer of soft paraffin to the chosen site so that the blood will not smear during sampling. Insert a disposable lancet about 2 mm and withdraw, cutting very slightly sideways. Wipe away the initial drop of blood with a dry cotton swab and then let the drops form and fall into the container. Squeeze and release your fingers around the calf to milk blood into the heel. Agitate the container to mix the blood with anticoagulant. When the required volume has been obtained wipe the heel and press with a clean cotton wool ball. This method is not suitable for obtaining blood for culture or for coagulation studies.

If the child or his mother are known to be at high risk of carrying hepatitis B or human immunodeficiency virus gloves should be worn and care taken to avoid needle stick injury to the operator.

1 Orlowski JP. My kingdom for an intravenous line. *Am J Dis Child* 1984;**138**:803.

Giving intravenous cytotoxics

J MIDDLETON

J LUKEN

C J WILLIAMS

Introduction

Since the introduction of anticancer chemotherapy three decades ago over 30 cytotoxic drugs have come into clinical practice. Although they may cure certain patients they may cause severe side effects; thus their use is best restricted to those experienced in cancer chemotherapy. As well as the harm that may be caused to patients by the injudicious use of cytotoxics, it should be remembered that they are potentially toxic to the hospital staff handling them. This chapter gives general advice on the correct ways of adminstering cytotoxics, though requirements vary according to the cytotoxics used.

Indications

Cytotoxic chemotherapy may cure some of the less common malignancies. But in many "solid" tumours its role is merely to prolong life. In such cases it is important to consider whether the potential therapeutic gain for the patient warrants the likely toxicity of the treatment. For palliative treatment the simplest (if possible oral) chemotherapy should be used and treatment stopped at the first sign of tumour progression or unacceptable side effects. When treatment is potentially curative every attempt should be made to reduce toxicity while maintaining intensive drug doses.

Contraindications

(1) Inadequate white blood cell or platelet count. Always check the results of a *fresh* blood count. Adjust the dose according to the recommended schedule for that drug regimen. Chemotherapy should be given in the event of pancytopenia only when the bone marrow is known to be affected by malignancy.

(2) Dysfunction of an organ which may be worsened by the cytotoxics to be used or which is the organ of excretion for that drug. For instance, bleomycin should not be

given when there is pulmonary damage that may have been caused by the drug; similarly, cisplatin, a renal toxic drug, should be avoided in kidney failure. To avoid such toxicity the doctor prescribing treatment should have an intimate knowledge of all the potential toxicities of each drug to be given. Monitor for potential toxicity and check relevant results *before* giving chemotherapy. Space does not permit a description of the likely toxicity of individual drugs; but organs that may be affected include the central nervous system, bone marrow, liver, kidneys, skin, mucosa, lungs, heart, and eyes. Inappropriate use of anticancer drugs may prove lethal. If you are not familiar with the drug you are about to administer ask someone who is.

(3) Known hypersensitivity—though some drugs such as bleomycin may be given with steroid cover.

(4) Infection is generally a reason for postponing treatment.

Equipment

Many anticancer drugs are given intravenously and the following equipment will be needed:
- An indwelling cannula; a 21 or 23 G butterfly needle is ideal for most situations
- Luer-Lok fitting syringes (to prevent accidental disconnection)
- Giving set with an injection port
- Intravenous solution (check compatibility with drugs to be administered)
- Hypoallergenic tape
- Sterile gauze to prevent leakage from connection contaminating the patient's skin and to cover the insertion site of the cannula after drug administration
- Gloves for the operator

Drawing up the drugs

Ideally the drugs should be drawn up by staff in a properly equipped pharmacy. There are well documented short term hazards of cytotoxic drugs and potential serious long term hazards (carcinogenicity and mutagenicity) which are being investigated. Precautions should be taken to protect the patient, operator, and environment. Current guidelines for drawing up and handling cytotoxics include:

(a) ideally, draw up cytotoxics in a laminar flow cabinet;

(b) wear gloves;

(c) use protective glasses;

(d) wear a mask when handling bleomycin, which comes as a dry powder in an ampoule;

(e) take care to avoid aerosol spraying—equalise pressure in rubber topped vials;

(f) clean up spillages immediately;

(g) protect the patient's skin from spillage.

Always check the compatibility of the drug, diluents, and intravenous solutions.

53

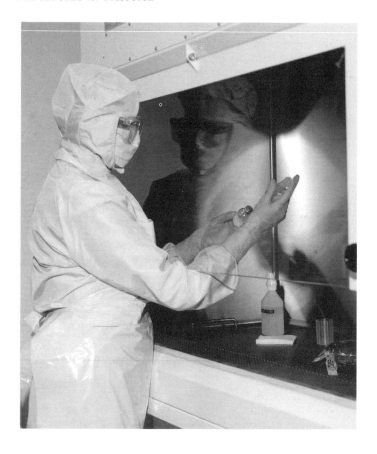

Procedure

Before starting to administer chemotherapy explain to the patient what you are going to do. Tell him about any side effects that may be expected and answer any questions he may ask. Try to ensure that the patient is in as pleasant and comfortable an environment as possible. Many patients will be frightened and a few minutes spent putting a patient at ease will make your job easier not only this time but during subsequent treatments.

Make sure that you understand the following important points concerning the drugs you are about to give:

(1) How to calculate the correct dose. Most cytotoxics are given according to the patient's surface area, which can be calculated from a nomogram using the patients current weight and height. Double check your calculation.

(2) Potential toxicities. Are there any contraindications to proceeding?

(3) Potential drug interactions.

(4) How quickly or slowly to inject the drugs: some drugs are unsafe when given as a rapid injection.

(5) Know what to do if the drug extravasates.

Make sure that the drugs are correctly labelled and that you have the right patient. *Never* give intravenous cytotoxics at the same time as intrathecal drugs: many cytotoxics are lethal if mistakenly given intrathecally.

Make sure that the patient is comfortable. It is usually best to have the patient sitting with his outstretched arm supported. Check that he is warm, so that his veins are distended; if a patient's veins are poor ensure that he sits with one arm in hot water for some time before treatment is given. Make certain that you are comfortable, sitting, and preferably not bending or kneeling. Always work in a good light. Check that there is an emergency call button and resuscitation equipment to hand.

If the patient already has a cannula in situ which you intend to use remove any dressings and check: (a) the patency of the vein and functioning of the cannula; (b) that there is no redness, swelling, or tenderness. Then, if you are certain that there are no problems, begin the procedure by flushing with isotonic saline (5–10 ml) and watch the vein carefully. But if you are in doubt it is safer to resite the cannula. When siting a cannula choose a large vein on the forearm, antecubital fossa, or dorsum of the hand. Never inject cytotoxic drugs into the veins of the leg. Use a sterile technique.

When the cannula is sited and properly taped down so that it is stable make sure of its patency and then inject the cytotoxic drug at the speed and in the manner recommended. If you are giving more than one drug use any vesicant drugs first, when there is the least chance of extravasation. Between each drug flush with 5–10 ml of isotonic saline. Watch the vein throughout so that you are aware of problems, especially extravasation, as soon as they arise. Involve the patient by asking about pain, discomfort, or abnormal sensation. Check for blood return frequently to ensure patency. If there is any sign of swelling or pain when a vesicant drug is injected *stop immediately*. Follow the recommended extravasation policy; do *not* continue. After injection flush with isotonic saline to prevent the drug from leaking from the puncture site.

Troubleshooting

Extravasation

Many cytotoxics are very vesicant and if they extravasate they may cause severe tissue damage. If, despite careful administration, extravasation does occur stop the injection immediately and follow the recommended policy in your unit. The following are general guidelines:

(1) Withdraw any drug by aspirating through the needle or cannula.

(2) Instil 50 mg hydrocortisone in 2 ml for injection into the site via the needle or cannula.

(3) Remove the intravenous device and instil a further 50 mg hydrocortisone in 2 ml subcutaneously into the swollen area.

(4) Resite the cannula well away from the area of extravasation and recommence drug administration.

(5) Advise the patient to take an analgesic, and ask him to contact the unit the following day so that you can check that there has not been a severe reaction.

Some investigators have recommended the use of hot or cold packs, hydrocortisone cream, and specific antidotes, but these remain controversial and their use is subject to local policy.

Local reactions

Redness and irritation sometimes develop along the vein being injected as a local reaction to the drug, especially when small veins are used. This may be reduced by further dilution, achieved, for example, by injecting the drug into a fast flowing infusion or injecting it more slowly. Intravenous hydrocortisone may be used at the end of the procedure.

Pain on administration

Some drugs (especially dacarbazine, vinblastine, and mustine) cause muscular and venous pain on administration. This pain is felt along the vein and not just at the site of the cannula, so is different from that caused by extravasation; further dilution or injection into a fast running infusion often helps.

Aftercare and complications

Nausea and vomiting

Many cytotoxic drugs cause severe emesis. It is therefore essential to make every attempt to achieve the best antiemetic control from the first treatment. Do not wait for the patient to vomit before starting antiemetics. If a patient does develop chemotherapy induced emesis conditioned vomiting rapidly develops. As well as ensuring good antiemetic cover try to make certain that the patient is as relaxed and comfortable as possible. Anxiety connected with cytotoxic administration seems to be related to the subsequent development of conditioned vomiting.

Other potential toxicities

Warn patients about other potential toxicities, in particular:

(1) *Bone marrow depression*—Ask patients to contact you if they become unwell, febrile, or have a possible infection. Patients with a potential infection should be seen *immediately* and a blood count should be performed. Sepsis during neutropenia is an emergency: patients can die within hours.

(2) *Stomatitis*—Patients should be advised about oral hygiene and should contact you if they develop severe ulceration or pain.

(3) *Cystitis*—The metabolites of ifosfamide and cyclophosphamide may cause a chemical cystitis and patients should be advised accordingly: fluid intake should be increased and, if necessary, mesna should be given.

(4) *Coloured urine*—Patients should be warned that their urine may become coloured for some hours after the administration of certain drugs.

Long lines

It is becoming more common to use tunnelled long lines from the start of intensive cytotoxic therapy. These should be inserted by an experienced operator under sterile conditions in an operating theatre. They are best maintained by a dedicated team who are used to dealing with such long term lines.

Infection of these lines in an immunocompromised host is a major hazard which may occur at insertion, later in the tunnel, or by colonisation of the catheter tip during a septicaemia. The following measures are necessary to minimise the risk of infection and keep the lines patent:

- Coordinate access to prevent a number of different people handling the line.
- Change the giving set every 24 hours.
- In the case of inpatients change the bung every 24 hours.
- Always use Luer-Lok connections to prevent air embolus.
- Use small gauge needles to inject through the bung.
- Ensure patency by flushing the line before and after use with either normal saline or heparinised saline.
- Avoid three way taps or extension tubing, both of which are a potential source of infection.
- Always use a strict aseptic technique.
- Re-dress site regularly using an aseptic technique.
- Teach the patient and relatives to handle the line; this adds to safety and reduces anxiety.
- Give the patient written information and a contact telephone number.

Caution

The administration and management of intravenous cytotoxic drugs are specialist tasks requiring extensive knowledge and practical experience about the pharmacology, toxicology, and effectiveness of these drugs. If you are in any doubt about their use ask someone experienced in cancer chemotherapy since these drugs are potentially lethal if misused.

Suturing

HAROLD ELLIS

Introduction

Suturing neatly and quickly is one of the important arts that should be acquired, as soon as possible, by a house surgeon or casualty officer. Even if he does not propose to pursue a career in surgery he will find this of value if his future lies in many other branches of medicine—general practice, anaesthesia, or even morbid anatomy.

Most suturing experience in the early days is connected with lacerations, and it is this aspect that will be dealt with here. The advice given also applies to closure of the skin in the operative wounds encountered in main theatre or after minor surgery in the casualty or outpatient department.

Contraindications

Small, superficial cuts will heal well if cleaned with a suitable detergent disinfectant, such as chlorhexidine, and covered with an adhesive dressing. This applies particularly to minor scalp lacerations within the hairline. Small children may not tolerate closure of a clean cut by sutures under local anaesthetic. Rather than submitting them to a general anaesthetic (and the subsequent trauma of having the sutures removed) their clean cuts can be disinfected, dried with spirit, and the edges apposed with Steristrips.

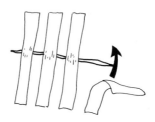

A small, clean wound closed with Steristrips.

If there is extensive skin loss, so that the wound can be apposed only under considerable tension, the tyro surgeon should call in a more senior colleague. Such wounds may need closure by mobilising a local flap of skin or, more commonly, by means of a skin graft—not to be attempted by the trainee.

Severely contused or heavily contaminated wounds (particularly when there has been a delay of six hours or more before surgery) should not be treated by primary suture because of the considerable risk of wound infection and breakdown. The wound should be cleaned and excised (as described below) and dressed with dry gauze. In the absence of infection delayed primary suture can then be performed on the fifth day with excellent prospects for satisfactory healing. A similar technique should be used in dealing with high velocity injuries—for example, gunshot wounds—in which, again, primary suture of the wound is likely to be followed by infection and wound breakdown. The only exceptions to this rule are contused or high velocity wounds of the head and neck. Here the magnificent blood supply of these tissues enables the surgeon to carry out primary suture with minimal risk of necrosis or infection.

Instruments and equipment

A very good rule, which cannot be learnt too early, is carefully to check all instruments and equipment before performing any operative procedure, no matter how minor this might be. This will obviate the embarrassment to the operator and the discomfort to the patient of such experiences as inserting a sigmoidoscope before making sure that the obturator can be removed or that the light will turn on.

Even for the relatively minor procedure of suturing a laceration there is quite an armamentarium to look over.

The instruments required are:
- scalpel handle size 3 with scalpel blades 10 and 15 (or a disposable scalpel)
- stitch scissors
- three to six fine artery forceps (depending on the extent of the wound)
- needle holder
- toothed dissecting forceps
- fine catgut for ligating blood vessels (3/0)
- fine nylon (3/0) swaged to a straight or curved cutting needle, depending on the operator's choice.

For local anaesthesia, 1% lignocaine with adrenalin, a disposable syringe, and disposable fine needles will be required.

For skin preparation either iodine *or* a detergent disinfectant solution such as chlorhexidine is needed.

In addition, the operator will require sterile disposable gloves, sterile dressings, sufficient sterile towels to drape the wound, Micropore to secure the dressings and, if the laceration affects the arm, a triangular bandage or a collar and cuff to use as a sling.

Before you start

A simple explanation of what you are proposing to do should be given to the patient (or, in the case of a small child, to the parents). If the wound is extensive, to any degree contaminated, or due to a perforation (for example, by a garden fork) consider the risk of clostridial infection. Check on the patient's tetanus immunisation and, if necessary, give a "booster" dose of tetanus toxoid. In all but perfectly clean lacerated wounds, start penicillin prophylaxis by intramuscular injection (use erythromycin in patients who are sensitive to penicillin).

Most patients can have their lacerations sutured by means of simple local anaesthetic infiltration. A particularly nervous patient may require a preliminary intravenous injection of diazepam in a dose of between 5 and 20 mg. A smaller dose is indicated in elderly subjects.

Procedure

In dealing with a lacerated wound the surgeon's aims are:

(a) to remove dead, devitalised tissue and any foreign contaminated material to reduce to a minimum the risk of wound infection;

(b) to stop bleeding;

(c) to approximate the skin edges (and, if necessary, the deep tissues) neatly and without undue tension to ensure as cosmetically favourable a result as possible.

A wide area of skin around the wound is carefully cleaned and then sterilised—for example, if the laceration involves the hand the skin from the forearm down to the fingers is prepared. If the skin is dirty it may need repeated scrubbing with soap and water. If hairy skin is involved a wide area around the wound is shaved and for this a disposable razor is particularly useful. Lacerations of the scalp should be widely cleared of hair; it is surprising how often an extension of the laceration or a second wound is discovered when blood stained, matted hair is cleared away.

Once the skin is clean, a wide area around the wound is disinfected with iodine or chlorhexidine and the area draped with sterile towels.

Local anaesthesia is achieved by infiltration with 1% lignocaine with adrenalin. If the initial injection is made within the lips of the wound, and if a fine needle is used, infiltration, even of the relatively extensive wounds, can be carried out almost painlessly.

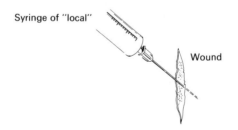

Syringe of "local"

Wound

Once the wound has become anaesthetised (and this is within seconds of infiltration) the lips of the wound are opened and the interior carefully explored. If there is an obvious spurting artery this is picked up at once with artery forceps. A large "spurter" may need to be tied off with 3/0 catgut. Small blood vessels can be treated by picking up with artery forceps, leaving the forceps on for a minute or two, and then twisting the forceps round and round before removing them. This torsion technique is very effective and saves burying a good deal of catgut in the wound. Scalp lacerations can bleed quite profusely. Here a useful technique is for the assistant to press firmly with the fingers on either side of the laceration down onto the scalp. Once the surgeon has sutured the wound the bleeding will cease simply as a result of the compression effect of the stitches.

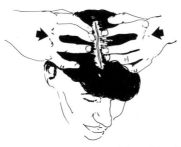

Pressure on the underlying skull on either side of a scalp laceration controls the bleeding.

A clean incised laceration needs no excision. In the case of contused wounds or crush injuries, the edges of the wound require excision back to healthy bleeding tissues. Usually the skin edges themselves require only minimal trimming with the scalpel (and this is particularly so in the highly vascular tissues of the scalp, face, and neck). However, the deeper tissues, particularly fat, should be excised more widely and the surgeon should ensure that only healthy, vascular bleeding tissue remains in the depths of the wound. Any foreign material (glass, fragments of clothing, road debris) must be carefully sought after and removed.

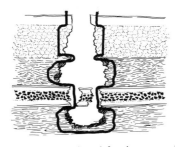

Remove all dead and foreign material.

It is the casualty officer or the house surgeon's duty to make sure what looks like a relatively minor wound does not conceal a more serious injury. In the case of a scalp laceration check that there is no underlying communication with a fracture. If the wound is over a joint make sure that the joint itself has not been opened; of course, lacerations of the wrist need careful preoperative and operative assessment to exclude injury to tendons, nerves, or major vessels. In any of these eventualities, send for help!

If the laceration is deep the deep tissues may need to be apposed with a few interrupted catgut sutures, and this applies also to the divided aponeurosis in a scalp laceration.

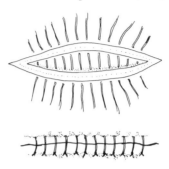

Simple sutures tied away from the edge of the wound.

Closure of the skin itself should be carried out, in most instances, by means of simple interrupted fine nylon sutures placed 2 or 3 mm from the skin edges. Sutures placed further from the skin edges simply result in ugly "cross hatched" scars. The knots should be positioned away from the skin edge and tied at just sufficient tension to appose the lips of the wound to each other. Tying the knots tightly simply strangulates the underlying tissues, whereas if the sutures are slack underlying fat tends to push out through the wound edges with a resultant ugly scar.

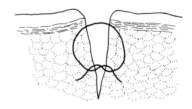

Fine catgut to appose the deep layers.

Mattress sutures should be used only if the surgeon finds difficulty in apposing the skin edges. Unlike the simple sutures, the knots here should be tied at the wound edge itself.

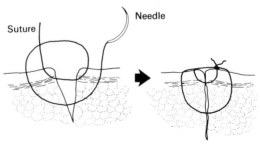

The mattress suture. The knot is tied at the wound edge.

The only other "fancy" suture that may be used is in the case of a triangular or Y shaped wound. The apex of the triangle is transfixed with a subcuticular stitch (as shown in the diagram) to prevent a gap at this point.

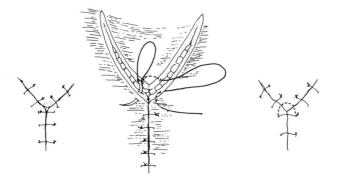

How to suture a Y or V laceration.

After ensuring that haemostasis has been achieved and that the wound has been neatly brought together, a dry dressing is applied and held in place with Micropore. In an extensive laceration of the hand do not hesitate to immobilise with a plaster front slab from the fingertips along the forearm. Similarly, an extensive laceration of the foot can be immobilised with a plaster back slab. A sling should be used in all arm injuries.

Aftercare

The patient should be provided with suitable oral analgesics and told to report at any time if the wound should ooze or become uncomfortable.

Sutures on the scalp, face, and neck heal with great rapidity and these can be removed in three or four days. The less time they remain, the neater the scar. When there is tension or when movement of the part may pull on the wound—for example, on the hand—the sutures should remain for 10 to 14 days—better a few days too long than to have the wound gape and require a secondary suture.

Ear syringing

STUART CARNE

Introduction

Wax (cerumen) is the secretion of the glands in the outer third of the external auditory meatus. Its consistency may be affected by atmospheric pollution. Normally it is expelled by ordinary chewing movements, but in some patients this does not happen. The wax then accumulates and may eventually block the external auditory meatus.

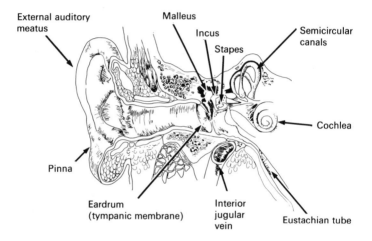

Indications

Symptomatic

(1) Hearing loss. (a) Acute onset: water in the ear may cause sudden swelling of the wax (for example, when swimming under water), which brings the patient rapidly to the doctor. (b) Gradual onset: the hearing loss may go unnoticed by the patient for a long time.
(2) Earache: when the wax is pressing on the drum.
(3) Cough: when the wax is pressing on the auricular branch of the vagus nerve.
(4) Giddiness: sometimes present when there is an obstruction by wax in one meatus only.

Asymptomatic

Wax is frequently seen on routine examination. If the examination is for an insurance or pre-employment medical it may be necessary to remove the wax to ascertain whether (a) the hearing is normal and (b) the drum is perforated.

Plugs of wax that do not block the meatus (and hence cannot affect the hearing) and still enable the drum to be seen may safely be left. Sometimes a thin film of wax on the drum (not painful) may give the impression that there is a perforation.

Note—The ordinary process of syringing when the middle ear is not inflamed often causes a temporary redness of the drum, which may confuse the diagnosis.

Contraindications

The presence of a perforation is a contraindication. Unfortunately, many patients are unaware of the perforation and it may not be identified until after the ear has been syringed. If necessary a prophylactic antibiotic should be administered systematically. Otitis externa is usually regarded as a contraindication because water can aggravate it. Nevertheless, many experienced doctors still syringe the ears when this condition is present but would always be careful gently to mop the meatus dry and might also instil some steroid drops (for example, betamethasone valerate lotion) twice daily for three or four days after syringing.

Wax in the ears of children poses special problems. Syringing the ears in a child is never easy and is particularly difficult when the child is ill; nor is the procedure free from risk of trauma, especially if the child is fractious. Many experienced practitioners prefer to treat the suspected diagnosis rather than risk physical and emotional trauma.

Equipment

- Syringe. Most ear syringes are about 18 cm long excluding the nozzle and hold about 120 ml of water (a). Shorter, but stouter syringes are available (b): though they hold less water they are easier to balance. A plastic syringe of this latter design is produced by Russell Instruments (PO Box 1, Clarkston, Glasgow G76). Some operators have found that a Water Pik (Teledyne Water Pik, Cranford, Middlesex), which is normally used in dentistry, is also useful for syringing ears. Alternatively, a Higginson syringe may serve the purpose. Whatever instrument is used, sterility is not necessary.

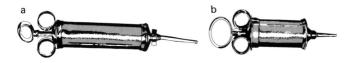

- Water. Plain tap water may be used and should be at or slightly above body temperature. The use of sodium bicarbonate in the water is not essential. Water that is too hot or too cold will stimulate the semicircular canals and may cause vertigo, nausea, and vomiting.

- Towels. Traditionally a rubber or plastic apron is wrapped round the patient's neck to protect his clothes. The cost of laundering cloth towels normally prohibits their use, but paper towels are a satisfactory substitute. They may be tucked inside the collar and will soak up most, if not all, of any water that spills.
- Collecting bucket. A Noot's tank is the most convenient, but if one is not available a kidney dish will do. The main disadvantage of the kidney dish is its habit of tipping over when partly full.
- Wax hook. A wax hook (Jobson–Horne) is useful to lift out a plug of wax that remains obstinately in sight but keeps falling back or one that is stuck to the side wall of the meatus. In most patients experienced operators can remove all the ear wax with a hook without recourse to syringing.
- Lighting. A source of light, either a battery auriscope or a lamp, speculum and head mirror, is essential for examining the ear before, during, and after the procedure. If a wax hook is to be used in the depths of the external auditory meatus a head mirror and speculum have an advantage over an electric auriscope in leaving one hand completely free to manipulate the hook.
- Wax softening agents. It is usually possible to syringe wax from an ear without any preparation, but first softening the wax eases the process. Sodium bicarbonate eardrops are effective. Alternatively, olive or almond oil or one of the proprietary preparations may be used. After any of these has been used for two to five days syringing may sometimes not be necessary. Some of the proprietary preparations, however, may cause otitis externa.

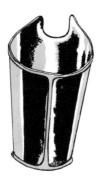
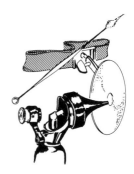

Procedure

If the indications for removing wax are not urgent prescribe a suitable solvent (for example, sodium bicarbonate) to be used in the affected ear(s) night and morning for two to five days and ask the patient to return at the end of that time. Alternatively, an immediate attempt to remove the wax may be made with a hook or by syringing the ear without preparation. There is some evidence that using a solvent solution for even half an hour before syringing may offer some benefit.

Have the patient sit comfortably in a chair, with his coat removed and a paper towel or plastic apron wrapped round his neck. The patient's cooperation is highly desirable if the meatus and drum are not to be damaged and water is not to be squirted all over the patient, the operator, and the rest of the room. Ask the patient to hold the Noot's tank below the ear, slotting the lobe into the groove. It is easier if the patient holds the tank to the right ear with the left hand and vice versa. This also reduces the risk of the patient knocking the operator's arm away.

When all is ready fill the syringe with water. Be sure no air remains in the syringe, as the sound of bubbles may be frightening to the patient. Pull the pinna up and back to straighten the external meatus. Put the tip of the nozzle at the edge of the external auditory meatus, pointed in the direction of the eardrum but slightly backward and downward (toward the patient's occiput). Some operators squirt the water in short bursts; others empty each syringeful in one or two actions. The jet of water should pass behind the wax and return into the tank. Sooner or later it will bring with it the lump of wax either intact or in fragments (often several large fragments: hence the need to inspect the ear during the procedure to ensure that all the wax has been cleared).

Water remaining in the meatus will restrict the view and should be gently mopped out with a pledget of cotton wool or paper tissue, but do not damage the eardrum in trying to make sure that the ear is perfectly dry. A small pledget of cotton wool may be left between the tragus and antitragus to mop up the last drops, but do not block the meatus.

When the first ear has been freed of wax turn the patient round slowly in his chair (rapid movement may make him giddy) and proceed in the same way with the other ear.

Complications

Even the most experienced operators sometimes fail to remove all the wax, even in the most cooperative patient and after using a softening agent. If the wax cannot be removed first time have the patient continue to use the softening agent for at least another seven days before repeating the procedure. If it again fails ask a more experienced operator to try; alternatively, refer the patient to an ENT surgeon. Rarely, a general anaesthetic may be necessary.

If the meatus is scratched it will bleed. This is particularly likely to occur if a wax hook is used by an inexperienced operator. The blood should be gently mopped up with cotton wool. Otitis externa is always a risk, but this may be reduced by careful drying (described above). If an already affected meatus is syringed the local application of steroid drops for one or two days after syringing reduces the risk of any further exacerbation.

Passing a nasogastric tube

A TUCKER

R M TERRY

Introduction

Passing a wide bore nasogastric tube is a routine nursing procedure: medical staff may need to intervene only when difficulty is experienced. Passing fine bore tubes carries more risk of perforation and should be performed only by medical or experienced nursing staff.

Indications

There are two main indications for passing a nasogastric tube. One is to aspirate stomach contents, either as a diagnostic test—for example, using pentagastrin—or as a therapeutic measure—for example, in the "acute abdomen." The other is to maintain nutrition of the patient, either when he should not swallow—for example, after pharyngeal surgery—or when he cannot swallow—for example, in postcricoid carcinoma, before treatment.

Contraindications

There are no absolute contraindications. Cuffed endotracheal or tracheostomy tubes should be deflated to allow passage of the tube.

Equipment

- Nasogastric tube. Choice of size depends on the purpose for which it will be used. Always use a large tube (say 16 FG) for aspiration: it is less likely to block during use or form a false passage during introduction. Large tubes may also be employed for feeding, but fine bore tubes (approximately 1 mm diameter) are preferable for this, as they are more comfortable for the patient.
- Lubricating jelly. Although a simple water soluble jelly (for example, K-Y) is usually used, lignocaine gel 2% antiseptic may be more comfortable for the patient, especially if the tube does not pass at the first attempt.
- Syringe (60 ml) for aspirating.
- Blue litmus paper to test the aspirated fluid for acid and confirm that the tip of the tube is in the stomach.

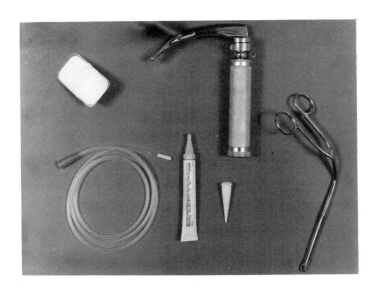

Before you start

Explain the procedure to the patient. Sit the patient well upright with head forward, if he is able to cooperate. Deflate a cuffed endotracheal tube in an intubated patient.

Procedure

A sterile technique is not required, although simple hygiene should be observed. Lubricate the nose with lignocaine jelly via the supplied applicator, and allow this to take effect. Gravity will assist the passage of the fluid to the back of the nose.

With the patient sitting, introduce the lubricated tube along the floor of the nose. Resistance will be felt as the tip reaches the nasopharynx: this is the least comfortable part of the procedure. Ask the patient to swallow (with a "feeder" of water if not contraindicated) as you continue to advance the tube, which should pass down the oesophagus without resistance. Never force the passage of any nasogastric tube.

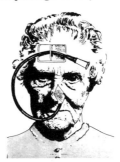

If a fine bore tube is being used never withdraw and reinsert the guide wire: always withdraw the entire tube and start again. At 40 cm in the adult the gastro-oesophageal junction is reached. Pass this and anchor the tube to the nose with reliable adhesive tape.

It is essential for the operator now to confirm the presence of the tip of the tube in the stomach. The most reliable method is to aspirate fluid and confirm that this is acid stomach content by a litmus paper test.

If no aspirate is obtainable (common with a fine bore tube) a radiograph to confirm the position of the tip will be required. Insufflation of air with simultaneous auscultation over the epigastrium is an additional confirmatory sign, but may still be positive if a viscus has been perforated.

In cases of doubt fluoroscopy or the use of a radio-opaque dye may be required.

Problems

Choking usually indicates the tube has entered the trachea and should be withdrawn immediately.

Difficulties in passing the tube may occur at any point along the route:

(1) *Nose*—Pass the tube along the floor of the nose and not towards the bridge. If one nostril is narrowed by a deviation of the nasal septum use the other side, although there is often a "tunnel" along the floor of the nose which can be used. In the event of persistent difficulty select a smaller tube and consider using a topical vasoconstrictor (for example, ephedrine 0·5% drops).

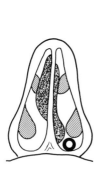 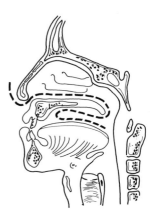

(2) *Oropharynx*—Reflex gagging by the patient may direct the tube into the mouth. There are various ways of dealing with this problem: try the following in order.

(a) Withdraw the tip into the nasopharynx and advance it again until you succeed in passing it into the oesophagus.

(b) Cool the tube in a refrigerator to stiffen it so that it is less likely to coil.

(c) Observe the passage of the tube through the mouth with a depressor on the tongue. Use a pair of long forceps (for example, McGill's) to guide the tube down.

(d) As a final measure, give the patient a benzocaine lozenge (10 mg) to suck for 10 minutes. Then lay him flat, remove the head of the bed, and use a Mackintosh laryngoscope to visualise the oropharynx. Direct the tube past the base of the tongue as an assistant introduces it through the nose. There is no need to visualise the larynx, for as long as the tube passes along the posterior pharyngeal wall it should enter the oesophagus.

(3) *Oesophagus*—A stricture or pharyngeal pouch may prevent the tube from passing and this is probably the only indication for a general anaesthetic.

Obstruction of the tube may be due to blockage by its contents or to the tube twisting on itself. A blockage should be cleared by flushing (citrate solution seems to help), and a twisted tube corrected by partially withdrawing it until it functions again, then relocating it.

The way the tube is fixed is important. If it is secured only to the cheek or forehead it may be accidentally removed if it is "caught" proximal to this.

Aftercare and complications

Wide bore tubes may need changing every four or five days if the patient's nose is sore.

Most fine bore tubes can be left in place for several weeks, but they have been known to coil in the stomach and re-enter the oesophagus.

Check the visible tube markings occasionally. Tubes can insidiously come out if there is traction on them, or the strappings come loose.

The main complications of the procedure arise from passage into the bronchial tree, or perforation of the pharynx or oesophagus. Failure to recognise these before the tube is used can be disastrous. The first fluid to be put down the tube should be sterile water.

The presence of an endotracheal tube does not preclude passage of the tube into the bronchial tree; peforation of the oesophagus is increased by the presence of oesophageal disease or cardiomegaly.

Laryngoscopy

PHILIP H BEALES

Introduction

Laryngoscopy is the method of examining the larynx from above by direct vision. It should always be preceded by inspection of the exterior of the larynx in the neck, carried out in a good light and with the patient's clothing removed. The larynx normally moves upwards on swallowing. In laryngeal stenosis the larynx moves downwards on inspiration, and it is immobile in tracheal stenosis. The patient should be seated and his head flexed when the larynx in the neck is palpated. The examiner stands behind the patient and palpation will disclose any broadening and tenderness that may indicate perichondritis of the thyroid cartilage. The larynx may be pushed forward in advanced postcricoid carcinoma. The larynx can normally be moved from side to side and a peculiar grating is often felt, which is normal and must not be mistaken for pathological crepitus.

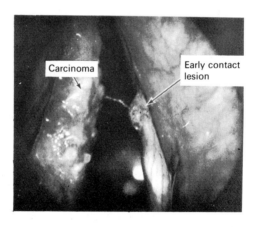

Indirect laryngoscopy

Indirect laryngoscopy is a diagnostic procedure only and no treatments or biopsies are carried out.

Indications

The commonest indications for indirect laryngoscopy, using a mirror, are persistent hoarseness; stridor; before thyroidectomy operations to establish normal vocal cord movements; dysphagia; earache; and to exclude a lesion, such as a carcinoma causing referred pain in the ear.

Contraindications

Contraindications are few, but the procedure cannot be performed in acute inflammations of the throat that give rise to trismus—for example, a peritonsillar abscess. Difficulty is experienced in young children, and direct laryngoscopy with an anaesthetic is usually required.

Equipment

- Laryngeal mirrors of different sizes
- A light source such as a good headlamp or a forehead mirror with a light source such as a bull's-eye lamp
- Pieces of gauze to hold the tongue
- A solution of 5% cocaine in a glass spray such as "Roger's crystal spray," or an amethocaine lozenge to be sucked before the examination
- Two stools, one for the examiner and one for the patient
- A mask for the examiner
- A spirit lamp for warming the mirror

Procedure

This is a simple procedure that is within the capabilities of every doctor who is willing to practise the technique; it should be performed more often that it is.

The patient is seated in front of the examiner, who sits at the same height. The examiner may wear a mask. It is important to explain to the patient what is to be done as his cooperation is essential. The patient sits upright with his head held level. The laryngeal mirror should be as large as possible. The light is directed onto the lips of the patient, who is asked to open his mouth and protrude his tongue as far as possible. His dentures must always be removed before the examination. The tongue is grasped between the thumb and middle finger of the examiner's left hand through the gauze swab. It is important not to pull the tongue too far forward or the frenum will impinge on the lower teeth and cause pain. The index finger of the left hand rests on the upper teeth to steady the hand.

The mirror is warmed over the spirit lamp, the flame being directed onto the glass surface. If a spirit lamp is not available hot water may be used. After the temperature of the mirror has been tested on the examiner's cheek, the mirror, held in the right hand, is introduced into the mouth and placed at the back of the uvula without touching the tongue, as this would smear the surface of the mirror. Steady pressure is maintained on the soft palate, and the light is directed onto the mirror. A reflection of the interior of the larynx will be seen, and the various structures may be examined in sequence by tilting the mirror. It is important to establish a regular routine of inspection in every case so that no details are missed.

The anterior surface of the epiglottis, the base of the tongue, and the valleculae are seen; and by tilting the mirror downwards and raising it the aryepiglottic folds, the false cords, the true vocal cords, and the upper tracheal rings can all be seen in turn. In the mirror image the vocal cords appear as flat, ribbon like structures with sharp, free margins. They are glistening white, and there should not be any visible blood vessels on their surface. The mobility of the cords should be observed during quiet respiration and by making the patient phonate by saying "ee." If there is no paresis or fixation the cords and arytenoids will approximate and the interarytenoid space will be obliterated. The subglottic space below the vocal cords cannot be seen, but, further down, the first two or three rings of the trachea may be seen anteriorly.

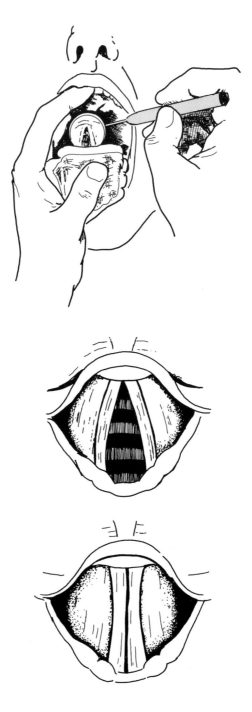

It should be remembered that the structures of the larynx are seen in a mirror; so the anterior part points away from the examiner and the right hand structures are seen on the left.

Difficulties

Some patients have an overactive "gag" reflex, and examination is difficult unless the soft palate is sprayed with an anaesthetic solution such as 5% cocaine or an amethocaine lozenge is sucked before the examination. It is often difficult or impossible to examine children by indirect laryngoscopy, but sometimes the larynx may be seen by placing the mirror almost horizontally against the hard palate, instead of the soft palate, so that the gag reflex is not excited.

The most difficult part to see is the anterior commissure, and it is vital for this area to be examined to exclude a carcinoma. Complete examination of the pyriform fossae is not possible by indirect laryngoscopy.

Direct laryngoscopy

Indications

Although in the past various manipulations such as laryngeal biopsy were done under indirect laryngoscopic control this is no longer the case and direct laryngoscopy is used for biopsy and laryngeal treatments. The method has been revolutionised by the development of microlaryngoscopy, which was first described by Kleinsasser in 1968. In this method the larynx is examined with a special wide laryngoscope held in position by a suspension system. The Zeiss operating microscope is used; it gives a magnified binocular view of the larynx. Fine instruments are available for accurate surgical treatment of such lesions as polyps and singer's nodes, and the biopsy of suspicious lesions. This is now the method of choice for treating lesions of the larynx endoscopically.

In recent years the carbon dioxide laser has been used for treating such lesions as pappiloma of the larynx and the removal of the early carcinoma of the larynx and vascular polypi of the vocal cords. The CO_2 laser is a new and powerful tool in endolaryngeal surgery.

Method

Under general anaesthesia with a hard, narrow bore catheter inserted through the mouth into the trachea the patient rests on his back with his head flexed against his neck and his teeth protected by a guard. When the muscles are relaxed the laryngoscope is inserted, and the structures in the vicinity of the larynx and the larynx itself are inspected so that all the structures are seen. The laryngoscope can be fixed in position by suspension attachments to the chest of the patient or the operating table, allowing the surgeon two hands to perform endolaryngeal surgery. The use of the binocular operating microscope in conjunction with direct laryngoscopy has become routine for most laryngoscopies.

Contraindications

Contraindications are few and would include injuries and diseases of the cervical spine, severe trismus, and appreciable laryngeal obstruction, when a preliminary tracheostomy may be necessary.

Complications

These are few and would include damage to the teeth and laceration of the lips and pharyngeal wall.

The photograph of the larynx is from Bull TR. *ENT Diagnosis*. London: Wolfe Medical, 1974.

Pericardial aspiration

A A GEHANI

R W PORTAL

Introduction

Pericardial aspiration is seldom indicated, and many doctors will neither have witnessed the procedure during training nor have performed it later in their careers. It is a potentially hazardous procedure and should not be performed except in emergencies unless facilities for resuscitation are available. Before inserting a needle into the pericardium there must be very good evidence that an effusion is present.

Indications

(1) As an emergency procedure to relieve cardiac tamponade.
(2) To obtain samples of pericardial fluid for analysis—for example, culture, cytology.

Pericardial puncture should *not* be undertaken to ascertain whether a pericardial effusion is present. Before embarking on the procedure carefully consider the evidence that an effusion (or haemopericardium) exists.

Diagnosis

Clinical signs

The physical signs of tamponade may be difficult to interpret, the chief alternative diagnosis obviously being cardiac failure from any cause. The picture of acute or progressive cardiac tamponade is one of circulatory embarrassment with tachycardia, raised jugular venous pressure, small pulse pressure, hypotension, muffled heart sounds, and pulsus paradoxus.

Pulsus paradoxus is elicited by allowing a very slow fall in sphygmomanometer cuff pressure while the subject breathes regularly and a little more deeply than normal. Occasionally the sign may be detectable on palpation of major pulses. The magnitude of the "paradoxus" is the difference in systolic blood pressure between the first hearing of the Korotkoff sounds on expiration only and the point at which they become continuous in both phases of respiration. (The term "paradoxus" is strictly a misnomer, for the phasic pressure difference is simply an exaggeration of the inspiratory fall in systolic pressure seen in normal subjects, but usually not readily detected.)

Remember that a pericardial rub is unlikely to be present with a sizeable effusion and that cardiac tamponade constituting an emergency cannot be present without raised jugular venous pressure.

Echocardiography

This is the most reliable method of proving a pericardial effusion and of assessing its volume or demonstrating loculation, but the M mode tracing or the two dimensional picture requires skilled interpretation. The ultrasonic beam will show a space between the pericardium and the anterior right or posterior left ventricular wall.

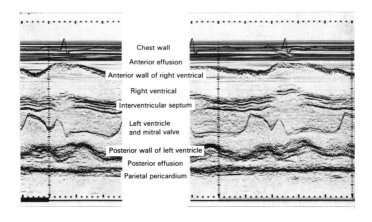

Chest wall
Anterior effusion
Anterior wall of right ventrical
Right ventrical
Interventricular septum
Left ventricle and mitral valve
Posterior wall of left ventricle
Posterior effusion
Parietal pericardium

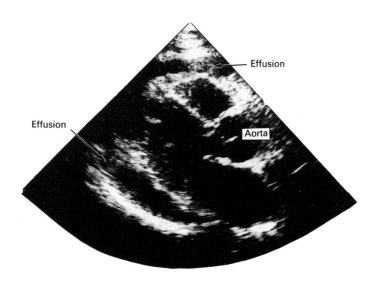

Effusion
Effusion
Aorta

Chest radiograph

In acute tamponade (for example, haemorrhage from trauma) the chest *x* ray film may show little or no cardiac enlargement. When time has permitted stretching of the pericardium the cardiac silhouette may be enlarged or grossly enlarged and appear pear shaped with bulging over the right atrium and apex.

The electrocardiogram

The ECG does not provide reliable evidence of pericardial tamponade or effusion. The presence of low voltage complexes should not be regarded as a specific diagnostic sign.

Contraindications

The main contraindication is doubt whether an effusion is present. After cardiac surgery (or possibly radiotherapy) loculation of fluid may increase the hazard of the procedure.

Equipment

- Sterilising fluid for skin (iodine, chlorhexidine)
- Sterile drapes
- Syringe and needles for injection of local anaesthetic (1–2% lignocaine)
- 18 G lumbar puncture needle
- Three way tap
- 50 ml aspiration syringe
- Spencer–Wells forceps
- Specimen containers

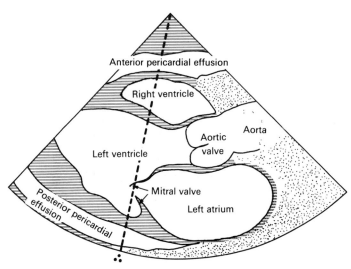

Triangular plane of corresponding M mode

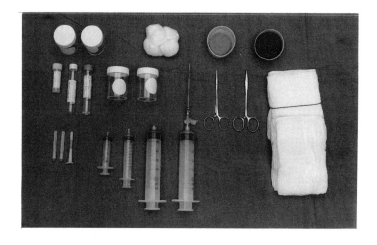

Before you start

Explain the procedure to the patient, who should be undressed to the waist and reclining comfortably in bed with thorax at an angle of 30–45° to the horizontal. He should be connected to an electrocardiograph (ECG) monitor, and an intravenous line or cannula should be inserted for administering drugs. If he is tense or anxious an intravenous injection of diazepam (perhaps 10 mg) will make the procedure easier for both patient and operator. The operator should wear mask, gown, and gloves. The skin at the site of puncture should be well cleaned and a sterile towel placed over the abdomen and legs.

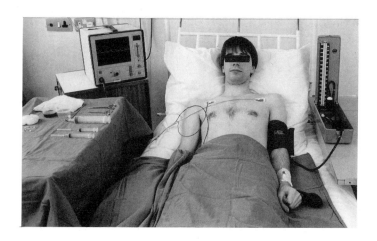

Procedure

Xiphisternal route

The safest and the recommended route is through the angle between the xiphoid process and the left costal margin. The skin and deep tissues are infiltrated with 10 ml of 2% lignocaine solution. The needle is aimed posteriorly at an

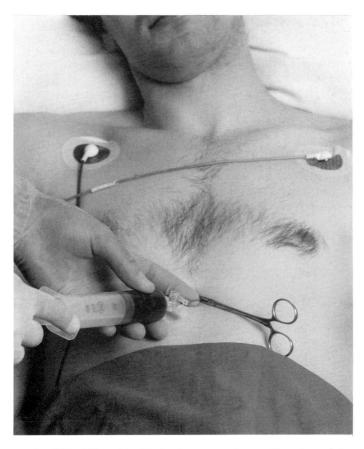

angle of 30–45° to the skin in the approximate direction of the left shoulder. The object is to traverse the membranous portion of the diaphragm opposite the middle of the diaphragmatic surface of the heart. The needle is advanced slowly, with gentle continuous suction, until the pericardial sac is entered and fluid is aspirated. Insertion of the needle some 5–7 cm (2–2½ in) will usually be required before the pericardium is reached.

The ECG monitor should be watched during insertion of the needle for the occurrence of ectopic beats or any other change. If the needle is advanced too far the myocardium will be felt knocking against the tip or will cause the needle to waggle. If this occurs withdraw the needle: never advance it further.

A Spencer–Wells forceps is clamped to the needle next to the skin to prevent further inadvertent penetration. By using the syringe and three way tap, fluid is aspirated; samples are sent for culture, cytology, and so on.

A bloodstained effusion may be distinguished from blood aspirated from the heart by placing a sample in a glass specimen bottle. A bloodstained effusion will not clot.

In cases in which repeated aspiration may be necessary a large needle may be used and a plastic cannula passed through this. The needle is then withdrawn, leaving the cannula in the pericardial space, secured to the skin with a stitch or plaster.

Apical route

The needle is introduced at the cardiac apex in the fourth or fifth intercostal space 2 cm medial to the lateral edge of cardiac dullness. This route carries a greater risk of injury to the coronary arteries and contamination of the pleural space when the pericardial fluid is purulent.

Parasternal route

The needle is introduced in the fifth left intercostal space just to the left of the sternum and aimed straight backwards. The internal mammary artery lies about 2 cm lateral to the sternal edge and the needle must pass medial to this: laceration of the artery is the main complication of this route.

Complications

- Vasovagal reaction (bradycardia, hypotension)
- Arrhythmias
- Laceration of ventricle
- Laceration of coronary artery
- Laceration of lung
- Laceration of internal mammary artery
- Spread of infection from a purulent effusion

Aftercare

The patient should remain on the ECG monitor for two hours after the procedure with observation of clinical condition, pulse, and blood pressure every 15 minutes. Any complication of the procedure is unlikely to become manifest after this period. A chest radiograph at this point is advisable.

Interpretation of results

(1) If tamponade is present clinical improvement may rapidly be observed after drawing off only 200–300 ml of fluid.
(2) An increasingly bloodstained effusion is a sign of needle trauma, so preserve the earliest aspirate for laboratory examination.
(3) A haemorrhagic aspiration is often present in malignant effusion and is to be expected in trauma.

Percutaneous central venous cannulation

M ROSEN

I P LATTO

W SHANG NG

Introduction

Central venous cannulation in surgical practice and intensive care has become more common with the impetus derived
from experience in cardiac surgery and developments in
disposable plastic catheters and cannulae. The procedure
may, however, result in serious hazard and even death. There
are numerous approaches to the central veins, and the
methods and equipment described here have been chosen as
those most likely to be safe and successful in the hands of an
inexperienced houseman called on to cannulate an adult
either breathing spontaneously or receiving lung ventilation.

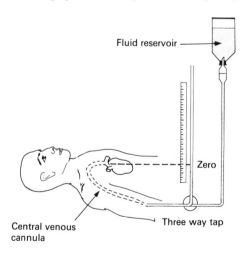

Fluid reservoir

Zero

Three way tap

Central venous
cannula

Indications and contraindications

Central venous pressure is the resultant of venous blood
volume, right ventricular function, and venous tone. Rapid
changes in blood volume, especially associated with impaired
right heart function, are the most common reason for monitoring central venous pressure. Pressures measured in peripheral veins cannot be relied on to reflect these changes.

Infusions of antibiotics, chemotherapeutic agents, and other substances irritant to veins and tissues are best administered through a line whose tip lies in a central vein. Potent drugs such as catecholamine solutions given at very slow flow rates are most reliably given through a central venous line. Drugs used in resuscitation of cardiac arrest should be given through a central line if one is available. In an emergency only a central vein may be accessible for administration of a rapid lifesaving infusion. This route is also widely used for long term intravenous alimentation. More sophisticated indications for central venous access include the insertion of a Swan–Ganz catheter and intracardiac pacing devices.

There are no contraindications to the method per se. Venepuncture should be avoided, however, at any site at which there is sepsis. Apical emphysema or bullae contraindicate infraclavicular or supraclavicular approaches to the subclavian vein. A carotid artery aneurysm precludes using the internal jugular vein on the same side. Furthermore, it may be wise to reconsider central venous cannulation in hypocoagulation and hypercoagulation states or if there is septicaemia.

Procedure

Sterility

Sterility should be maintained during the insertion of the cannula. The skin should be carefully cleaned—for example, with 0·5% chlorhexidine in 70% alcohol (Dispray 1 Quick Prep (Stuart Pharmaceuticals Ltd) is a convenient form)— and sterile towels applied round the site. The operator should wear a mask, gown, and gloves, and in an emergency gloves at least should be worn. Although some catheter systems are designed to be used ungloved, in practice contamination may sometimes occur through an error or technical difficulty. A small (5 cm³) syringe and heparinised saline such as Hepsal (Weddell Pharmaceuticals Ltd) which contains 10 IU/ml heparin in normal saline are useful for flushing the line as soon as it is inserted.

Equipment

(1) Catheter through cannula. This type of device is recommended for inserting a long catheter through an arm vein. A well designed example is the New Drum Cartridge Catheter (Abbot Laboratories Ltd). A cannula on the outside of a needle is placed in the vein and the needle withdrawn. A catheter is inserted through the cannula and is then threaded into the vein. When the catheter is in position the cannula is withdrawn.

(2) Catheter over needle. In an arm vein the needle and the catheter are placed in the vein, the needle (which is attached to a wire) withdrawn, and the catheter advanced into position. A shorter version of this is the long cannula over a long needle (100–150 mm) which is intended for use in the internal jugular and subclavian veins. A safety

feature in some of these devices is a means of occluding the hub to prevent bleeding and air embolism—Wallace Flexihub (Medical Assist (Anglia) Ltd), Secalon T (Viggo).

(3) Catheter through needle. This is the simplest method and was once widely used. It has been condemned because improper use may result in the catheter being sheared off. Most manufacturers have withdrawn this type of apparatus.

(4) Catheter over guide wire. A flexible guide wire is inserted into the vein through a needle. After removal of the needle the catheter is inserted over the wire, which guides it into the vein. This technique is recommended as a safer alternative to the long cannula on long needle method for internal jugular and subclavian vein catheterisation since probing for the vein is carried out with a short small bore needle. Complete kits are available— Leader-Cath (Vygon (UK) Ltd). A guide wire with a J shaped tip increases successful catheterisation of the external jugular vein—Hydrocath (Viggo).

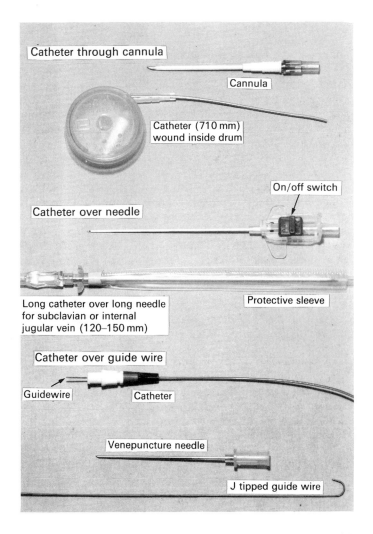

A stylet is useful to thread the catheter forward and to indicate the length of catheter in the patient. The presumptive position of the tip can be estimated and the catheter withdrawn if necessary so that the tip lies above the nipple line. A precoiled catheter (inside a drum) can be more frequently placed in the superior vena cava.

Methods

The techniques are described in order of safety and effectiveness. In each, air embolism is avoided by maintaining the venous pressure above atmospheric by position or a tourniquet on the limb. If the patient is conscious the skin should be infiltrated with a local anaesthetic using a fine needle.

Arm veins

The median (basilic) arm veins are the safest approach to the central venous system. The cephalic vein curves sharply to join the axillary vein through the deep fascia at the shoulder, which may impede passage of a catheter. This results in less successful central placement, but it is still worth attempting. The veins are distended by a tourniquet. The head is turned to the same side to compress the neck veins, and the arm is abducted. The catheter should be of 600 mm minimum length. When the tourniquet is released air embolism may occur, so depress the proximal end of the catheter below the level of the patient's elbow.

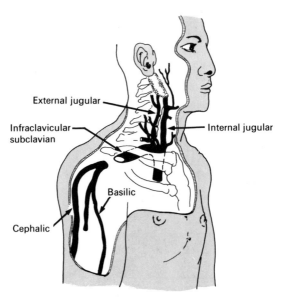

External jugular vein

The external jugular vein runs from the angle of the mandible to behind the middle of the clavicle and joins the subclavian vein. The patient is placed in a 20° head down position with the head turned to the opposite side. The most prominent vein is chosen. If neither vein becomes visible or palpable cannulation is inadvisable. In about half the attempts the catheter cannot be threaded into an intrathoracic vein, but successful central placement may be helped by digital pressure above the clavicle, by depressing the shoulder, or by flushing through the catheter. The use of a Seldinger wire or a spiral J shaped wire increases the incidence of successful central placement of the catheter. The use of excessive force should be avoided. Satisfactory measurement of central venous pressure is sometimes possible from the external jugular vein or from the junction of the external jugular and subclavian veins. This junction is a common site for the distal tip to lodge when the catheter will not thread centrally.

Internal jugular vein

The internal jugular veins run behind the sternomastoid close to the lateral border of the carotid artery. The vein may be cannulated with a low incidence of major complications by an approach well above the clavicle. The patient is placed in a 20° head down position with the head turned to the opposite side. The right side is preferred to avoid injury to the thoracic duct and is also easier for the right handed operator. The sternomastoid muscle, cricoid cartilage, and carotid artery are identified. With the other hand the carotid artery is palpated and protected at the level of the cricoid cartilage. The needle is attached to a saline filled syringe and inserted just lateral to the artery. The needle is directed towards the feet parallel to the midline with the syringe raised 30° above the skin. Gentle aspiration is maintained as the needle is advanced. A flush of blood into the syringe signifies entry into the vein. For operators of limited experience these steps should be first carried out using a small (21 G) needle to locate the vein before proceeding with the larger bore cannula, using the small locater needle as a guide. If the artery is punctured use firm compression for five minutes.

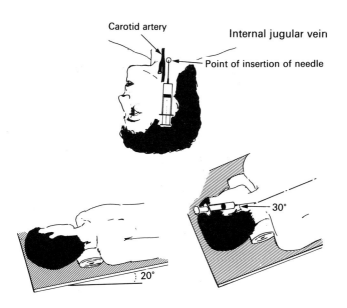

Infraclavicular subclavian vein

The subclavian vein is particularly suitable for administering long term parenteral nutrition. It is widely patent even in states of circulatory collapse, so that subclavian venepuncture may provide the only route for rapid infusion. Puncture and catheterisation of the subclavian vein is a blind procedure. Serious harm can be inflicted on nearby vital structures, and deaths have been reported. The most common complication is pneumothorax. The procedure, therefore, should not ordinarily be performed by an inexperienced operator without close supervision. The subclavian vein lies in the angle formed by the medial one third of the clavicle and the first rib, in which the subclavian vein crosses over the first rib to enter the thoracic cavity. There is some variation in the anatomy of this region, which has prompted the use of an ultrasound probe to facilitate locating the position of the subclavian vein. This manoeuvre, however, is unlikely to reduce the incidence of pneumothorax. The patient rests supine, tilted 20° head down. Either side may be used, although the right side is preferable. The patient's head is turned to the opposite side. The midpoint of the clavicle and the suprasternal notch should be identified. The distance between the skin puncture and the vein necessitates using a long needle and cannula. The needle is attached to a saline filled syringe and inserted below the lower border of the midpoint of the clavicle. The needle tip is advanced close to the undersurface of the clavicle, aiming at the suprasternal notch. While the needle is advanced gentle aspiration should be maintained, and a flush of blood indicates that the vein is entered. If the attempt is unsuccessful, further attempts may be made, altering the direction of the needle only when it has been withdrawn to just beneath the skin. A chest radiograph should always be taken to check for pneumothorax.

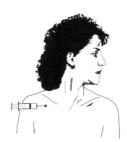

Infraclavicular subclavian vein

Diameters of needles or cannulae and lengths of catheters recommended for each route of insertion

Route of insertion	Outside diameter of needle or cannula	Minimum length of catheter (mm)
Arm vein	14 G	600
External jugular vein	16 or 14 G	200
Internal jugular vein	16 or 14 G	150*
Subclavian vein	16 or 14 G	150*

*Long cannulae are available (120–150 mm long, 14–18 G o.d.).

Checking and testing

Blood should be aspirated to ensure that the catheter is in a vascular space before injecting fluid. If the line is connected to a bottle of fluid that is lowered below the patient blood should flow freely under the influence of gravity. On connection to a column of fluid for measurements of central venous pressure the fluid column should show slow oscillations related to respiration and quicker oscillations related to the heart beats. A chest radiograph should be taken to confirm that the position of the tip is above the right atrium, preferably not more than 2 cm below a line joining the lower borders of the clavicles.

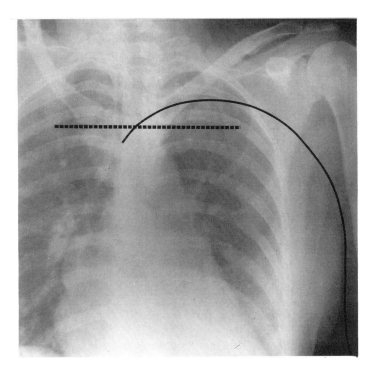

Management

Fixing the catheter

Once satisfactorily placed, the catheter should be fixed carefully to prevent inadvertent withdrawal or movement further into the vein. Firm fixation probably also reduces the

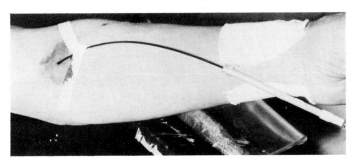

89

incidence of thrombophlebitis. Adhesive tape (1 cm width) is crossed over to grip the catheter firmly, away from the venepuncture site. An alternative, especially for longer term use, is to secure the catheter with a skin suture.

Asepsis

The most scrupulous attention to detail is needed to keep venous catheters infection free. Strict aseptic technique during the insertion of the catheter is essential. Additions to intravenous fluids should preferably be introduced in the aseptic laboratory of the pharmacy. The intravenous giving set should be changed daily, an aseptic technique being used while connecting it to the catheter. Injecting drugs into the venous catheter and taking blood samples through stopcocks should be avoided if possible. Regular bacteriological monitoring of the venepuncture site should be carried out. It is important to be vigilant to detect catheter related infections. If an infection occurs the catheter should be removed immediately.

Clotting

It is important to maintain a continuous flow through the catheter to prevent reflux of blood and clotting. After making intermittent measurements of venous pressure, using a simple manometer filled with saline solution, it is a common fault to forget to turn on the infusion again, resulting in a catheter blocked by a clot. It may be possible to clear the catheter by injecting 2–5 ml heparinised saline under pressure.

Complications

Complications of central venous catheterisation mostly fall into two categories—firstly, those that occur at the time of catheterisation and result from injury to some vital structure; and, secondly, those that occur at a later stage and are associated with catheter related thrombophlebitis and infection. In addition to these two groups air embolism, catheter embolism, cardiac arrhythmias, and perforation of the myocardium may occur at any time. Suspicion should be aroused if there are unexplained cardiovascular disturbances. Perforation into the mediastinum or pericardium may be recognised only on a routine chest radiograph. An offending catheter should be withdrawn to a safer position and any infusion stopped. Timely application of a tourniquet may prevent a sheared off catheter migrating up an arm vein. A catheter embolus requires early intervention for its removal. Disturbances of cardiac rhythm stimulated by a catheter in the heart usually subside spontaneously but, if not, the catheter should be withdrawn into the superior vena cava. Persistent severe arrhythmias require urgent treatment. When arm or external jugular veins are used serious immediate complications are rare. The veins are usually visible and palpable. Catheters lying in peripheral veins, however, often lead to thrombophlebitis if left in position for more than one or two days. Most immediate and serious complications are a feature of blind venepuncture of the subclavian and, to a lesser extent, internal jugular veins. Injury to many structures related to the thoracic inlet has been reported: pneumothorax, haemothorax, arterial puncture, and damage to the thoracic duct and phrenic nerve. The need for insertion of a chest drain will depend on the size of the pneumothorax and the respiratory embarrassment it causes. Drainage is required if the pneumothorax is 50% or more. If smaller, observation of the patient and a repeat chest radiograph in 4–6 hours (more frequently in patients on positive pressure ventilation) will reveal an increasing pneumothorax. A tension pneumothorax requires immediate drainage with a small bore needle. A haematoma in the neck associated with arterial puncture is usually controlled by applying firm pressure for five minutes. Close observation of the site should be continued. Surgical repair is only rarely needed. The complication rates reported after catheterisation of the deep veins range between zero and 15% and are probably dependent on the experience of the operator.

Immediate	Immediate or later	Later
Arterial puncture	Air embolism	Myocardial perforation
Cardiac arrhythmias	Catheter embolus	and tamponade
Injury to thoracic	Pneumothorax	Hydrothorax
duct		Infection
Injury to nerves		Venous thrombosis

Pleural aspiration and biopsy

P B ILES

COLIN OGILVIE

Indications

Pleural aspiration may be used to help make a diagnosis, to relieve symptoms from a large effusion, or to instil therapeutic agents, such as antibiotics, cytotoxics, or sclerosants, into the pleural space. It can prevent effusions—especially those which are purulent or haemorrhagic—from becoming chronic and thus avoid the development of pleural thickening and a "frozen chest." It is sensible to perform pleural biopsies with the first aspiration since this increases the diagnostic yield and because there may be insufficient pleural fluid remaining on later occasions to permit a safe biopsy.

Contraindications

Because the commonest complication of pleural aspiration or biopsy is pneumothorax, either from puncture of the visceral pleura or from air entry through the chest wall or apparatus, the presence of severe bullous emphysema or severe obstructive airways disease is a relative contraindication, especially when the effusion is small. The risks are less and benefits greater with a large effusion. Impaired clotting—for example, in liver disease—may also be a contraindication to biopsy. There is a recognised risk of seeding mesothelioma cells in the biopsy track and therefore if this disease is suspected from the history or clinical features it is wiser to reserve biopsy for those patients in whom pleural fluid cytology has not been diagnostic.

Equipment to put on trolley

Pleural aspiration
- Sterile gloves, gown, and towels
- Dressing pack with cotton balls, gauze swabs, galley pots
- Skin antiseptic
- Syringes: 10 ml and 50 or 60 ml (Luer-Lok fitting)
- Hypodermic needles: 21 and 25 G (several of each)
- Lignocaine 2%: 2 × 10 ml ampoules
- Pleural aspiration pack with needles or trocars and cannulae (various sizes)

92

or
- E–Z Cath intravenous placement unit (12 or 14 G)
- Three way tap
- Rubber tubing
- Receiver for fluid
- Scalpel blade
- Adhesive dressings

Pleural biopsy
- As above
- Abrams needle
- Skin suture pack and Spencer–Wells forceps

Specimen bottles
- Fluid: (1) 3 × 20 ml sterile plain bottles for microbiology, biochemistry, and serology; (2) bottle with anticoagulant for cytology; (3) oxalate bottle for glucose
- Biopsy: sterile dry bottle, or one with saline for microbiology and formal saline for histology

Drugs: for example, antibiotics, cytotoxics, sclerosants.

Before you start

Order in advance from the pharmacy any drugs which are to be instilled into the pleural space—for example, cytotoxics, irritant immune stimulants such as *Corynebacterium parvum*, or agents for pleurodesis such as tetracycline.

Check that anticoagulated containers for cytology specimens are available. Ask the histology laboratory whether pleural biopsies are preferred in saline or in formalin.

Review the most recent posteroanterior and lateral chest radiographs and re-examine the patient to decide the proposed site for the procedure—for example, lateral or posterior. If in doubt about whether there is effusion or consolidation lateral decubitus radiographs, or preferably an ultrasound examination, should resolve the uncertainty and may also identify the height of the diaphragm.

Aspiration procedure

It is important that the patient is as comfortable and relaxed as possible; some explanation of what he will feel during the procedure should be given. The patient should be positioned leaning slightly forwards with his arms folded comfortably before him and resting on a pillow. He may be either seated facing the side of his bed with his arms on it, or in bed with a bed table as support for his arms. When the fluid is not loculated the easiest site for puncture is on the posterior chest wall medial to the angle of the scapula, one interspace below the upper limit of dullness to percussion. A common error is to insert the needle too low down or too far forward.

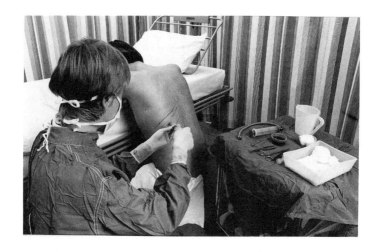

The operator should scrub up and be gloved and gowned as for any surgical procedure. The patient's skin is prepared with a suitable antiseptic and sterile towels. The skin overlying an intercostal space at the chosen level is infiltrated with 1% or 2% lignocaine using a 25 G (orange hub) needle. This is then changed for a 21 G needle (green hub) to infiltrate the chest wall down to the pleura. When the needle penetrates the pleura fluid should appear in the syringe as the plunger is withdrawn. To avoid damaging the intercostal neurovascular bundle the inferior border of the upper rib is avoided. Care must be taken to ensure that air does not enter the pleural space at any stage of the procedure.

When the tap is for diagnosis only 20–50 ml fluid is aspirated into a fresh sterile syringe and put into the appropriate containers.

To remove a large quantity of fluid use a needle with attached three way tap or a ready prepared pack consisting of needle, three way tap, connecting plastic tubing, syringe, and collecting bag. Aspirating large volumes of fluid in this manner may be protracted and uncomfortable for the patient, and it is sometimes easier to insert a catheter such as the 12 or 14 G E–Z Cath intravenous placement unit and, after withdrawing the central needle and stylet, to connect a three way tap and syringe to the Luer-Lok fitting on the end. When the needle or catheter is removed a small adhesive dressing is adequate for the puncture site.

Patients with empyema and haemothorax

Difficulties may arise in patients with empyema and haemothorax when the fluid is thick or loculated. Aspiration may be possible only with a large bore needle, and exploratory aspiration at several different sites may be necessary. The finding of pus is an indication for instilling antibiotics while the needle is in the empyema space; it may be difficult to locate the space at a later attempt. If the empyema is a complication of a bacterial pneumonia then laboratory information on the organism and its antibiotic sensitivities may already be available to guide the choice of antibiotic. If this guidance is not available then ampicillin (500–1000 mg) in

10–20 ml of water for injection or a cephalosporin should be instilled. Pus that smells foul usually indicates an anaerobic infection, for which oral or parenteral metronidazole is appropriate. Repeated aspiration and intrapleural instillation of antibiotic should be continued until pus is no longer obtainable. If there is then still evidence of continuing infection insertion of an intercostal drainage tube is indicated, followed, if necessary, by rib resection with evacuation of the empyema cavity.

Biopsy equipment

The Abrams needle is the one most widely used in Britain for pleural biopsy. A Cope needle of the blunt type may be more suitable when little or no pleural fluid is present, and the Tru-Cut needle is usually reserved for biopsies of consolidated lung. The Abrams needle consists of outer and inner tubes, the outer acting as a trocar. Behind the tip of the outer tube is an opening into which a fold of pleura is to be impacted. This opening is closed completely when the cutting edge of the inner tube is advanced by twisting its hexagonal grip clockwise. This rotation moves a pin in the hilt of the inner tube forwards along a spiral slot in the hilt of the outer tube. The biopsy specimen is cut by the sharp advancing edge of the inner tube and is retained within the instrument. It can then be retrieved by using the accompanying blunt obturator.

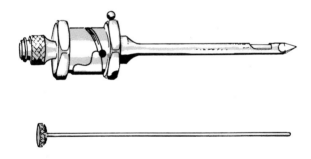

Biopsy procedure

Position and prepare the patient as for a pleural aspiration, and infiltrate the intercostal tissues at the chosen site generously with lignocaine. It is important to check that fluid can be aspirated into the syringe; note also the approximate thickness of the chest wall down to the pleura. Make a short (3–5 mm) incision through the skin and continue with blunt dissection, using the Spencer–Wells forceps, through most of the chest wall thickness. The closed Abrams needle is then introduced through the tissues and parietal pleura with a slight rotary movement. Connect a three way tap and syringe to the Luer-Lok fitting on the needle, rotate the hexagonal hub on the inner tube anticlockwise to open the notch and aspirate pleural fluid in the usual manner. The needle is normally airtight when the notch is closed but a syringe or closed three way tap must be attached when the notch is open to prevent air entering the pleural cavity.

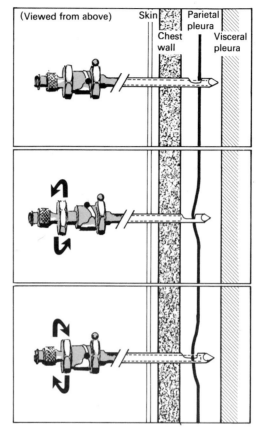

When taking a biopsy specimen it is convenient to have a small (2 ml) syringe attached to the needle. Rotate the grip to open the notch, which faces the same direction as the spherical marker on one facet of the hexagonal hub of the outer tube. With this marker (and therefore the notch) facing along the line of the intercostal space (to the left if the operator is right handed) apply lateral pressure towards the notch with the forefinger and slowly withdraw the needle until resistance is felt owing to pleura catching in the notch. If the needle is withdrawn too far only intercostal muscle will be obtained. Hold the needle firmly and sharply twist the grip of the inner tube clockwise to take the specimen. Withdraw the needle with a slight rotary action when the patient exhales, covering the entry site with a gauze swab as the needle emerges. To avoid damage to the intercostal neurovascular bundle the notch should never be directed upwards. The specimen will be found either within the inner tube or in the tip of the needle and should be put in 10% formal saline. It is best to take three or four specimens if possible. If tuberculous pleurisy is suspected some of the pleural biopsy specimens should be taken and placed in a dry sterile container for bacteriological culture.

Troubleshooting

Failure to obtain any fluid

The commonest error in cases of difficulty is to insert the needle too low down or too far forward. If uncertain try higher. If the pleura feels unusually thick and the needle moves through a wide arc on respiration it is probably in the diaphragm.

No fluid may be present—for example, there is consolidation or marked pleural thickening. The value of ultrasound in identifying fluid in this instance has been discussed.

The fluid may be very viscous, as in empyema or haemothorax. Use of a needle of wider bore may be successful.

Loculated effusions

If only a small quantity of fluid is obtained the collection may be loculated. Ultrasound can demonstrate the loculi and the most promising aspiration sites marked on the chest wall; or the aspiration may be performed in the *x* ray department with further ultrasound guidance as necessary.

Specimens

Pleural fluid for microscopy and culture should be collected in a clean dry sterile container and transferred to the laboratory as soon as possible. Containers with anticoagulant are necessary for cytological examination. For biochemical analyses the same bottles as those used for blood samples are satisfactory. The use of pots containing formalin for histological examination of biopsy specimens and dry pots for microbiology has been discussed.

The more relevant the information given on laboratory request forms—for example, bacterial pneumonia, asbestos exposure, contact with tuberculosis, etc—the more useful the laboratory results are likely to be.

Aftercare and complications

It is wise to obtain a chest radiograph after pleural aspiration, particularly if any difficulty was experienced—air drawn back into the syringe or a large volume of fluid obtained. It is essential after pleural biopsy or if the patient experiences chest tightness or bouts of coughing.

If fluid is removed too quickly or in too great a quantity oedema may develop in the re-expanded lung tissue. It is usually recommended that not more than 1·0–1·5 l is aspirated at one time, although in small patients even 700 ml may be the limit. If the lung is unable to re-expand freely a high negative intrapleural pressure may develop as fluid is aspirated. This will be felt by the operator as an increased pull on the syringe plunger and by the patient as chest tightness accompanied by coughing. Both of these complications can be relieved by letting air into the pleural space to lower the negative pressure, but this delays re-expansion of the lung and may permit loculation of the fluid.

In the absence of a clotting defect pleural aspiration rarely leads to serious haemoptysis or haemothorax. The former may occur if pleural biopsy is attempted without first obtaining fluid and the latter if the vessels at the lower border of the rib are damaged. Pneumothorax can result if the needle tip penetrates the visceral pleura or if air is inadvertently allowed to enter via the needle. If the pneumothorax is large an intercostal drain with underwater seal may be required. If the aspiration needle tears the visceral pleura and a superficial vein air may be sucked into the pulmonary veins from the needle itself or from the adjacent lung. The air may enter any systemic artery, most often the cerebral vessels, and produce transient neurological symptoms and signs. The customary emergency treatment is to tilt the patient's head down and with his right side uppermost to reduce the chance of air entering these arteries. Many deaths previously certified as "pleural shock" were probably due to air embolus, but vagal inhibition can also occur. Empyema after a non-sterile aspirating technique is rare, but nevertheless infection may be introduced and convert a sterile pleural effusion into a difficult empyema. Possible complications in cases of mesothelioma have already been mentioned.

Thoracoscopy

This technique has usually been performed under general anaesthesia by thoracic surgeons but has now become a physicianly procedure too, carried out under local anaesthesia and using a fibreoptic bronchoscope in place of a rigid thoracoscope. Details of the method are beyond the scope of this chapter, but it is the most reliable way of obtaining a positive pleural biopsy specimen.

Interpretation of results

The table shows the pattern of results most frequently seen; but, inevitably, it is incomplete.

The following points are worth remembering. Protein levels may not distinguish between exudates and transudates. The limit of detection of leucocytes by microscopy is one cell per high power field; this is roughly equal to 1×10^7 cells/l. Coulter counters can give more accurate results, although high fibrin content in pleural fluid may cause measurement problems. A shimmering satin sheen to pleural fluid indicates the presence of cholesterol in a chronic effusion but gives no clue to the cause.

Guide to results of laboratory tests on pleural fluid

Condition	Appearance	Protein concentration (g/l)	White cell count	Predominant cell type	Cytology	Histology	Culture	Other features
2° to infection	Clear or cloudy	> 3	+	Polymorphs	Negative	Negative	Negative (usually)	
Empyema	Cloudy or purulent	> 3	+ + +	Polymorphs	Negative	Negative	Positive	Offensive smell with anaerobes
Tuberculosis	Clear or cloudy	> 3	+ or + +	Lymphocytes	Negative	Positive	Positive (occasionally)	
Pulmonary infarct	Clear or bloody	> 3	+	Polymorphs or eosinophils	Negative	Negative	Negative	
2° malignancy: pleural involvement	Bloody or clear	> 3	+	Variable	Positive	Positive (often)	Negative	
altered fluid turnover	Clear	> 3	± or +	Polymorphs	Negative	Negative	Negative	
Mesothelioma	Clear or bloody	> 3	+	Variable	Positive (usually)	Positive	Negative	
Trauma	Clear or bloody	> 3	+ or + +	Polymorphs (eosinophils occasionally)	Negative	Negative	Negative	

Guide to results of laboratory tests on pleural fluid (*continued*)

Condition	Appearance	Protein concentration (g/l)	White cell count	Predominant cell type	Cytology	Histology	Culture	Other features
Connective tissue disorders	Clear or cloudy	>3	+ or ++	Variable	Negative	Negative	Negative	
Rheumatoid arthritis	Clear	>3	+	Variable	Negative	Negative (rarely positive)	Negative	Very low glucose; rheumatoid factor positive
Cardiac failure	Clear	<3	± or +	Variable	Negative	Negative	Negative	
Hypoproteinaemia	Clear	<3	±	Variable	Negative	Negative	Negative	
Chylothorax	Milky	>3	±	Lymphocytes	Negative	Negative	Negative	Microscopic fat globules

± = 0–2 leucocytes/high power field.
+ = <5 leucocytes/high power field.
++ = <15 leucocytes/high power field.
+++ = >15 leucocytes/high power field.

Kidney biopsy

PAUL SHARPSTONE

RICHARD McGONIGLE

Introduction

Patients with renal glomerular disease may present with similar clinical features yet have conditions ranging from trivial to life threatening. Their prognosis and treatment depend on the renal pathology, and histological examination of the kidney is often the only way to make the diagnosis. Needle biopsy provides a sample of perhaps 20–30 of the 2 000 000 glomeruli and so is unhelpful and may give misleading results in patchy conditions such as reflux nephropathy. It is most valuable in assessing and, in particular, indicating the prognosis of patients with diffuse glomerular disease.

Principal indications

Clinical syndrome	Indications for biopsy
Asymptomatic proteinuria	Protein excretion more than 1 g/24 h Red blood cells in urine Impaired renal function
Haematuria—macroscopic and microscopic	Urography and cystoscopy do not show source
Acute nephritic syndrome	Persisting oliguria
Nephrotic syndrome	Adults: unless cause is apparent from extrarenal manifestations. Children: only if haematuria also present, or if proteinuria persists after trial of corticosteroid
Acute renal failure	No obvious precipitating cause Obstruction of the renal tract excluded
Chronic renal failure	Radiographically normal kidneys
Renal allograft	To differentiate rejection from cyclosporin toxicity, and to diagnose recurrence of original disease

Contraindications

Laceration of the kidney may cause haemorrhage, which may lead to nephrectomy. The risk is small but should always be kept in mind, and biopsy should be done only if the other kidney is adequate. A single kidney or major abnormality of the contralateral kidney are contraindications, as is any haemorrhagic tendency, including advanced uraemia. The platelet count should be over $100 \times 10^9/l$ and the prothrombin time should give an International Normalisation Ratio less than 1·3. Biopsy should not be done on shrunken kidneys because they are difficult to locate, the histological findings are often non-specific, and, in any case, the result is unlikely to provide information of any therapeutic relevance.

Equipment

- Tru-Cut disposable biopsy needles (Travenol Laboratories Ltd): 11·4 and 15 cm
- Exploring needle: 17 cm, 1·1 mm (19 G)
- Scalpel blade: No 11
- Syringes: 10 and 2 ml
- Needles: 21 G (green) and 25 G (orange)
- 1% lignocaine: 10 ml
- Diazepam injection (Diazemuls): 10 mg/2 ml
- Skin disinfectant
- Sterile gloves, towels, and swabs
- Bath towel

Before you start

Check the patient's blood pressure, blood urea and creatinine concentrations, haemoglobin, platelet count, and prothrombin time. Send blood to the laboratory for "group and save." Make sure that an intravenous urogram has been done and that films are available. Arrange a mutually convenient time for performing the biopsy between the operator and the radiologist who is to conduct the ultrasound examination. Check that the time is suitable for the histology technician to attend with a dissecting microscope. Explain the procedure to the patient and have him practise holding his breath in inspiration. Biopsy is unsafe if he cannot cooperate. Obtain his informed consent in writing.

Procedure

Renal biopsy is potentially hazardous, and the inexperienced should do it only under skilled supervision. Premedication with intravenous diazepam makes the procedure less unpleasant for the patient; general anaesthesia is required only for infants and young children. A firm surface is needed, and to "fix" the kidneys roll up a towel (about 10 cm in diameter) and put it under the patient's abdomen between the rib cage and pelvis. Place the patient prone with his head turned away (most patients do not want to watch), his arms abducted, and his forearms beside his head.

Although the use of intravenous urography to locate the kidneys in relation to bony landmarks has served well for many years, we now prefer ultrasound imaging at the time of biopsy. The site of choice is the edge of the lower pole of the left kidney. This avoids major renal vessels and is likely to contain more cortex than medulla. The radiologist marks it on the skin and tells you the depth of the kidney there. Nevertheless, except in patients with end stage renal failure and in transplanted kidneys, always have an intravenous urogram done first to ensure the patient has two functioning kidneys with no gross anatomical abnormality.

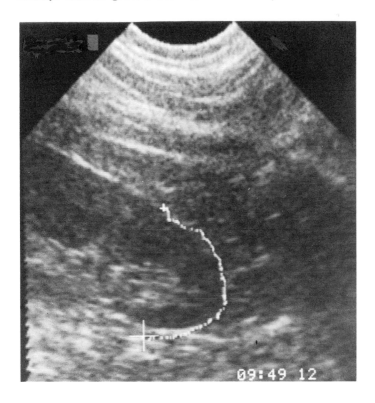

Wear sterile gloves and stand at the left side of the patient. Prepare the skin and locally anaesthetise the skin and subcutaneous tissues; then use an exploring needle to find the kidney. Insert it into the lumbar muscles and then advance it 5 mm at a time until a definite swing with respiration shows that the point is within the kidney. Ask the patient to hold his breath in inspiration each time you move the needle and to breathe out and in after each advance. Do not restrict movement of the needle while the patient is breathing: handle it only while he is holding his breath. After locating the kidney, inject local anaesthetic along the track while withdrawing the needle.

The 11·4 cm Tru-Cut needle is suitable for most patients but use the 15 cm one for larger patients. Make a nick in the skin with the point of a scalpel blade and then advance the biopsy needle, with the cannula closed over the obturator, stepwise as with the exploring needle. A large arc of swing usually shows that the kidney has been located, but beware the patient who uses his chest more than his diaphragm when asked to breathe deeply. When the swing is small it is easy to penetrate the full thickness of the kidney, and the specimen obtained will comprise only fat or blood clot. In these patients correct location of the point of the needle depends on feeling the resistance of the capsule and the "give" on penetrating it. The disposable needle is sharp and the change in resistance slight; so, for sensitive control, hold it low down by the shaft rather than by its handle. A small jerk with each respiratory movement means that the tip of the needle is just scraping the capsule and should be advanced a little further. If the needle moves only at the extreme of inspiration it is probably being struck by the lower pole and should be reinserted higher up.

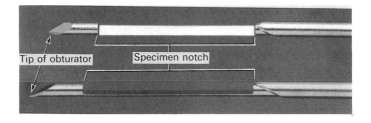

When you are satisfied that the tip is *just* within the kidney ask the patient to hold his breath in inspiration. Then tap the obturator handle in, push the cannula smartly down the length of its travel to cut the specimen, keeping the obturator handle firmly fixed with the other hand, and finally withdraw the needle with the cannula closed over the obturator. The last three manoeuvres must be made while the patient is holding his breath, so practise them on a ripe pear first.

Troubleshooting

A successful biopsy produces a strip of kidney up to 20 mm long. The various histological techniques require the specimen to be divided into at least three portions, so examine

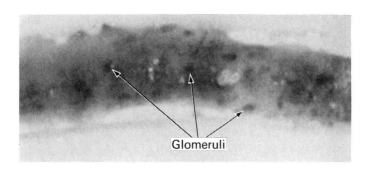

each with a dissecting microscope and make sure that all contain glomeruli. If there is any doubt about their adequacy obtain another specimen rather than risk having to repeat the whole performance later on when you receive the histology report reading "medulla only."

The specimen

Immunofluorescent microscopy is carried out on fresh tissue while routine, immunoperoxidase, and electron microscopy require appropriate fixatives. Consult the histopathology laboratory about its requirements or, preferably, arrange for a technician to collect the specimen.

Make sure to include on the request form details necessary for a helpful interpretation of the histology such as the patient's age, blood pressure, renal function, amount of proteinuria, multisystem disease, and drug history.

Aftercare and complications

The patient should remain in bed for 24 hours and have his pulse and blood pressure checked every hour for four hours and then every four hours.

The most important complication is haemorrhage, which may be perirenal, causing loin pain and sometimes a palpable mass as well as the signs of blood loss; or intrapelvic, causing persisting heavy haematuria and sometimes clot retention. More minor haematuria is common and usually settles quickly. Continuing haemorrhage should be treated by blood transfusion and sedation and, if necessary, selective embolisation after arteriography to locate the source. Exploration of the kidney is only rarely required.

Interpretation of results

Even the most experienced and skilled renal histopathologist cannot give all the answers, even in diffuse glomerular disease; and remember the sampling error in focal lesions.

Liver biopsy

J R F WALTERS

A PATON

Introduction

Percutaneous needle biopsy of the liver is a simple bedside procedure that provides a core of tissue for laboratory investigation and so is valuable in many types of liver disease and systemic illness. Several different instruments are available, each with its own technique. The general principles apply to all, but our discussion of procedure is confined to the disposable Tru-Cut needle. Liver biopsy may also be carried out at laparotomy and laparoscopy and transvenously, but we do not propose to discuss these methods.

A blind procedure in an organ as vascular as the liver can be hazardous, so physicians should be well prepared and rehearsed. Practice with the appropriate instrument may be got in the necropsy room, but there is no substitute for learning by watching and copying someone who performs liver biopsies every week.

Indications

(1) Confirmation of a clinical diagnosis of cirrhosis.
(2) Investigation of chronic hepatitis and assessment of the effects of treatment.
(3) Histological confirmation of primary and secondary tumours.
(4) Investigation of "difficult" jaundice.
(5) Investigation of the effects of drugs, including alcohol, on the liver.
(6) Occasionally in acute hepatitis and hepatomegaly, and when liver function tests give abnormal results that remain unexplained.
(7) As an aid to diagnosing pyrexia of undetermined origin, granulomatous disease, and lymphomas.

Contraindications

Can the patient understand the procedure and hold the breath for five seconds? A violent cough or gasp when the needle is in position may tear the liver, with disastrous bleeding. A general anaesthetic is usually required in children.

Is the patient likely to bleed excessively? The prothrombin time is the best indication: if it is prolonged more than three seconds and biopsy is considered to be essential then fresh frozen plasma should be given (one unit before, one during, and one after the biopsy); if it is over six seconds the procedure should not be carried out. When the prothrombin time is abnormal 10 mg of vitamin K may be given parenterally for a few days. The platelet count is less important, but if it is below $50 \times 10^9/1$ ($50\,000/mm^3$) care should be taken; platelet concentrates may be used.

Is the path to the liver normal? Biopsy is best postponed when there is a skin or chest infection. Ascites causes the liver to float away from an advancing needle and when appreciable should be treated first.

Is biopsy likely to do more harm than good? Patients with deep jaundice, especially from extrahepatic obstruction, where the bile ducts are dilated, risk biliary peritonitis as well as haemorrhage, and if cholangitis is present the infection may be spread. Biospy should only be undertaken by those with considerable experience. Consider the possibility of a hydatid cyst, when anaphylaxis may result, or a vascular tumour including hepatoma, when angiography may be a better investigation.

Equipment

Check the trolley before you start and lay out the equipment, if possible away from the patient's bed. There should be:

- Plenty of cotton wool and gauze swabs
- Three or four sterile towels or drapes
- A small bowl for methylated spirits (we prefer not to use iodine)
- A 10 ml syringe for local anaesthetic
- A selection of hypodermic needles

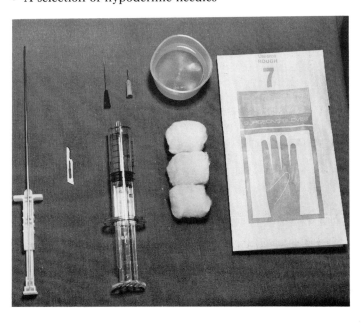

Lay out the Tru-Cut needle after testing the movement of the trochar and cannula. A small scalpel blade will be needed, and we like to have a 22 G spinal needle with which to measure the depth of the liver. A pair of sterile diposable plastic gloves should be provided.

Before biopsy

Make sure the patient understands the procedure and has given informed consent.

Specimens of blood will have been sent to the laboratory for a full blood count, including platelets, prothrombin time, blood grouping and cross matching of one pint of blood, and standard liver function tests.

Ultrasound examination is helpful, especially when the liver is thought to be shrunken by cirrhosis or where bile ducts may be dilated by obstruction.

No restrictions need be placed on the patient's eating or drinking.

Procedure

The patient lies along the edge of the bed with the right arm behind the head, which is turned to the left. A pillow placed firmly along the left side of the body will keep it horizontal. Palpate the abdomen and percuss the liver in the mid-axillary line: remember that it is largely intrathoracic. Mark the rib space which is below the top of the liver dullness on full expiration. It may be helpful to mark the xiphisternum and liver edge as well.

Sedation is not usually necessary, but plenty of local anaesthetic is. Draw up 10 ml of 1% lignocaine. Clean the

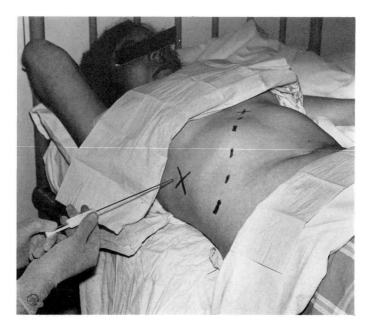

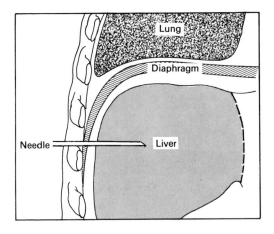

skin with methylated spirit, and anaesthetise through a 25 G needle with a few drops of lignocaine in the appropriate space just above the rib. Then, using a 21 G needle, anaesthetise the deeper tissues with the patient breathing quietly, and advance slowly until a scratchy sensation or a gasp of pain indicates the sensitive tissues overlying the liver. Infiltrate this area with large amounts of anaesthetic. Remove the needle and, if you wish, measure the approximate distance to the surface of the liver on the biopsy needle.

Instruct the patient on how to take several deep breaths in and out and how to hold the breath in deep expiration for as long as possible. When you are satisfied with the manoeuvre nick the skin with the point of the scalpel blade, introduce the biopsy needle, and advance slowly with the patient breathing quietly. If you are not sure of the depth of the liver surface continue advancing cautiously until the needle begins to swing with respiration, then withdraw slightly until it stops swinging.

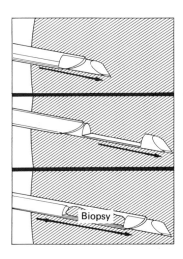

Repeat the breathing instructions with the patient following you. As soon as the breath is held in expiration thrust the *closed* needle about an inch into the liver. Advance the inner trocar, holding the outer cutting sheath still. Fix your right elbow against your side (to prevent the instinctive desire to withdraw the needle), advance the outer cutting sheath to cut the liver in the biopsy notch, and quickly withdraw the whole needle from the patient. With practice this sequence should take only a second or two. We prefer it to the one recommended by the manufacturer, as do others we have consulted, because it ensures that the specimen is taken from within the liver rather than from under the capsule.

Cover the skin incision with a plaster and instruct the patient to lie on the right side for four hours and to remain in bed for 24 hours. Pulse rate and blood pressure should be recorded hourly, and nurses instructed to report at once any alteration in condition or any complaint of pain.

The specimen

Remove the biopsy specimen from the notch and divide it if specimens are needed for bacterial culture, biochemical examination, or electron microscopy in addition to histological examination. Place the histological specimen in 20 ml formol saline on a piece of card to prevent fragmentation. Record the procedure in the notes, together with the texture of the biopsy specimen and its appearance to the naked eye: fat, pigmentation, tumour, and cirrhosis can sometimes be recognised. Do not forget to note time of procedure, any instructions, and who to contact in the event of complications.

Complications

No liver tissue is obtained—This occurs most commonly when the sequence of movements is incorrectly performed, the inner trocar being withdrawn when the outer sheath should have been advanced. Incorrect positioning (as in very fat people, when it may be difficult to outline liver dullness), inadequate expiration, or a small or mobile liver are other reasons. The experienced performer permits no more than two attempts at biopsy.

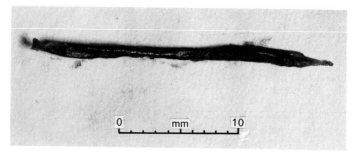

Severe pain may be caused by bleeding or leakage of bile. Pain in the shoulder tip and discomfort over the site of biopsy when the effect of the local anaesthetic wears off may require simple analgesia. Anything more than this should always be reported and patient and nurses instructed accordingly. Biliary peritonitis is fortunately rare.

Shock is usually caused by rapid loss of blood from a large vessel or vascular tumour, less often by Gram negative septicaemia. Bleeding may be more insidious, and blood transfusion should be started if there is unexplained tachycardia or hypotension, and fresh frozen plasma or platelets given if indicated.

Septicaemia may result from needling an infected bile duct or liver abscess and may be the first indication of infection.

Rarer complications include haemoptysis or pneumothorax owing to biopsy of the lung, and biliary or bacterial peritonitis owing to puncture of gall bladder or colon respectively.

Anything more than slight pain or discomfort should be treated promptly and more serious complications must be considered an emergency. Consult a surgeon early. Though fortunately rare, death can occur from haemorrhage or biliary peritonitis, and delayed laparotomy contributes.

Tapping ascites

G NEALE

Introduction

The detection of fluid in the peritoneal cavity (ascites) always indicates serious disease. At least 500 ml must be present before it is possible to detect the classical signs of fullness in the flanks, shifting dullness, and a fluid wave. If the patient can get on to his hands and knees smaller volumes of fluid gravitating to the periumbilical area may be percussed as a circle of dullness. If there are doubts examination by ultrasound is a simple, useful technique capable of detecting small quantities of fluid and demonstrating localised

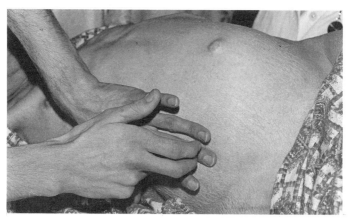

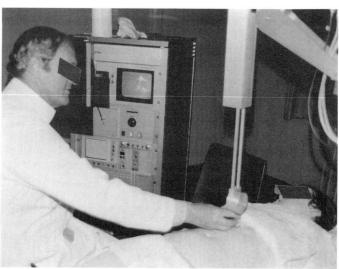

collections. Sometimes ascites is diagnosed when none exists, especially in patients whose viscera are filled with fluid (for example, fluid in loops of small intestine or in large, lax ovarian cysts), and, conversely, may not be detected when it is localised by peritoneal attachments.

Table I—Causes of ascites

Associated with chronic disorders

Common causes
Cirrhosis of the liver
Abdominal cancer
Tuberculous peritonitis
Heart disease (especially constrictive pericarditis)

Rare causes
Liver disease without cirrhosis
Hepatic vein occlusion
Severe hepatitis
Chronic pancreatic disease
Myxoedema
Chronic renal disease
Polyserositis (for example, systemic lupus erythematosus)
Other inflammatory conditions (for example, Crohn's disease)
Ovarian disease

Associated with acute abdomen

Bacterial peritonitis
Trauma (haemoperitoneum)
Acute pancreatitis
Strangulated viscera (especially intestine)

In the neonate (extremely rare)

Renal abnormality (with leakage of urine)
Intestinal abnormality (for example, obstruction with perforation)
Cardiac failure
Cirrhosis
Infection (for example, toxoplasmosis)

Indications

Tapping ascites

Tapping ascites is a simple, safe procedure for which the indications are as follows: (1) to investigate the cause of ascites and when necessary to take a specimen of peritoneum for biopsy; (2) to assess bacterial infection of ascitic fluid; and (3) to treat by (a) removing fluid to relieve abdominal discomfort or severe dyspnoea or (b) introducing chemotherapeutic agents.

Tapping the abdomen is used principally as an aid to diagnosis. It is a vitally necessary investigation in the patient with possibly infected ascites (usually in association with longstanding chronic liver disease). In patients at risk, unexplained fever, a raised white cell count, or a general deterioration (often with signs of encephalopathy) are warning signals which should not be ignored. With modern diuretics it is only occasionally necessary to drain ascites to relieve severe discomfort or secondary dyspnoea. In some liver units fluid removed from the abdomen of a patient with cirrhosis and resistant ascites is ultrafiltered and reinfused into a systemic vein to prevent severe protein depletion.

Tapping the acute abdomen

Paracentesis is not used universally to investigate patients with acute abdominal disorders even though many reports over the past 50 years have extolled its value. It is used when the diagnosis is in doubt, especially after abdominal trauma. The site of puncture is determined by the local clinical findings. If there is generalised abdominal tenderness tapping in the four quadrants of the abdomen may be performed followed by needling the flanks. Local anaesthesia is usually unnecessary for this procedure. If the tap yields no fluid and there is still doubt about the diagnosis it may be worth attempting to aspirate fluid from the pouch of Douglas. This is done by inserting a dialysis catheter through the linea alba, and some doctors believe that peritoneal lavage using this technique may be helpful.

Indications for the procedure are as follows: (1) puzzling diagnostic problems, especially in those regarded as presenting high operative risks; (2) obtunded patients in whom there are signs suggesting intra-abdominal disease (especially after trauma); and (3) suspected non-surgical acute abdominal disease (for example, pancreatitis).

Apart from contraindications (see below) there are special considerations when needling the acute abdomen. Analysis of fluid obtained either directly or by lavage should not be relied on if the results are inconsistent with other findings. The procedure is probably most usefully performed when one doctor in the hospital takes special responsibility for the investigation and its interpretation.

Taking a peritoneal biopsy

Biopsy of the peritoneum is useful in diagnosing non-purulent ascites in which the fluid has a protein concentration of over 25 g/l, is not rich in amylase, and in which direct examination does not show malignant cells nor acid fast bacilli.

Contraindications

There are no absolute contraindications to tapping ascites. Provided sterile methods are used and a few precautions taken, passing a fine needle into the peritoneal cavity is totally safe even when fluid cannot be aspirated. The removal of large quantities of fluid is rarely necessary. If performed the patient should be examined four or five times over the next 36 hours to check for signs of hypovolaemia, consequent oliguria, or hyponatraemia.

Special care must be taken in handling instruments and aspirated fluid when treating patients who have viral hepatitis, in whom there is circulating hepatitis B antigen, or who may carry the virus causing the acquired immune deficiency syndrome.

Much more care needs to be taken when needling the acute abdomen. In general, paracentesis should not be carried out on: (1) patients in whom the diagnosis appears to be clear cut or in whom a diagnosis may be achieved by non-invasive investigations; (2) patients with multiple scars and distended bowel; (3) patients with localised inflammatory disease (results are usually unhelpful); and (4) pregnant patients.

Equipment

Ascites may be tapped quite safely with a simple, sterile technique using a fine needle on a syringe. If there are likely to be difficulties in finding fluid or if the operator wishes to obtain 100 ml of fluid or more (which may require more than one needle puncture) then it is wise to have a trolley with the following equipment:
- Dressing pack
- Sterile skin cleaning fluid
- Various needles (long 19–23 G are the most useful)
- Various syringes (5 ml for local anaesthetic; 50–100 ml for aspiration)
- Local anaesthetic (1 or 2% lignocaine)
- Abrams biopsy needle (for description see Pleural aspiration and biopsy, p. 92)
- Catheters (12 or 14 G), connecting plastic tubing and collecting bag (if considerable quantity of fluid to be removed)
- Specimen containers

Preliminary arrangements

Tapping ascites may be undertaken on a couch in the clinic or at the patient's bedside. If difficulties are expected—for example, small quantities of loculated fluid—the procedure may be best performed under scanning control. It is necessary to ensure that the appropriate laboratories are ready to receive specimens and that the local arrangements are followed. For example, the cytologist usually specifies desirable quantities of fluid in citrated bottles delivered direct to the laboratory.

Next the procedure needs to be explained to the patient and his agreement obtained. The patient is asked to go to the toilet to empty his bladder. This serves two purposes. Firstly, one wishes to avoid passing a needle into a distended bladder, and, secondly, the change in position may disperse cells which have sedimented in the peritoneal cavity after prolonged bed rest.

Procedure

The procedure may be undertaken as follows.

Ask the patient to lie relaxed in a supine position. Re-examine the abdomen and select a site for puncture. (Usually this site will be in an area in which there is shifting dullness and under which there appear to be no solid organs. The iliac fossae, away from the inferior epigastric blood vessels and scars, are the areas most often used, and it may be helpful for the patient to roll slightly to the side of the operation to maximise the area of dullness. Aspiration through the less vascular linea alba is occasionally used for therapeutic procedures and before laparoscopy.)

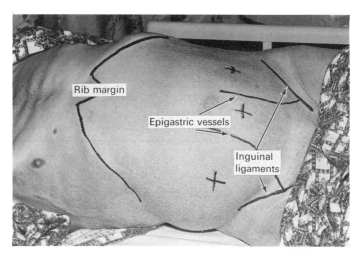

Put on a mask and sterile gloves. Clean the skin and infiltrate 3–6 ml of local anaesthetic into the anterior abdominal wall down to the parietal peritoneum. Attach a long, fine needle (19–23 G) to a large syringe and introduce the needle into the abdominal cavity. (Often a sense of give is felt in passing across the anterior and posterior fascial layers and, to a lesser extent, in perforating the peritoneum.) Aspirate gently. Fluid will flow easily into the syringe if the tip of the needle is correctly placed. If no fluid is obtained reposition either the patient or the needle. Remove up to 50 ml of fluid, withdraw the needle, and apply a simple dressing to the skin. In patients with suspected tuberculosis it is worth taking much larger quantities of fluid and using the centrifuged deposit to isolate the causative organism.

A peritoneal biopsy may be undertaken after demonstrating the presence of free fluid. Remove the exploring needle and introduce an Abrams punch through a small skin incision. Attach the punch to a syringe and open the notch by twisting the hexagonal grip anticlockwise. Aspirate a little fluid. Angle the open notch against the peritoneal surface and withdraw the punch slowly until it engages the abdominal wall. Twist the hexagonal grip clockwise and withdraw the punch. Remove any tissue from the edge of the notch and, if necessary, repeat the procedure (it is virtually impossible to obtain tissue when the peritoneal surface is normal).

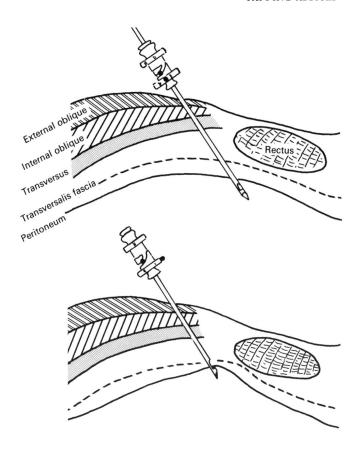

Troubleshooting

The procedure is usually trouble free. Problems occur most often in obese patients with minimal quantities of fluid. A "dry" tap may indicate failure to enter the peritoneal cavity, perforation of a viscus, or occlusion of the end of the needle with a piece of omentum. The inexperienced operator should reposition the tip of the needle and continue to aspirate on withdrawing the needle slowly. If necessary he should seek help from a more experienced clinician. It is reasonable for that person to make two attempts on each side of the abdomen. If no fluid is obtained the abdomen should be scanned to determine whether or not the diagnosis of ascites is correct and to indicate how best to approach a small quantity of loculated fluid.

Specimens

The appearance of the fluid removed by tapping the abdomen should be noted. A cloudy fluid often means peritonitis; uniform bloodstaining is most often found in patients who have cancer or who have suffered trauma to the abdomen; and a milky fluid indicates chylous ascites.

117

Aliquots of the fluid are sent to the laboratory for cytological examination, cell count, measurement of protein concentration, and, in selected cases, enzyme estimations and bacteriological culture. Details of the patient's illness and of the clinician's specific request must be included on the laboratory form. The specimens will be handled individually and the quality of examination will depend on the knowledge and skill of the pathologist. Direct discussion is often very helpful in resolving difficult problems and in determining how much weight to give to the result of the laboratory investigation.

Aftercare and complications

Tapping ascites rarely leads to complications. Inadvertent puncture of the intestine is rare, and even if intestinal contents are aspirated secondary infection is most unusual. The management is conservative although it is necessary to check the temperature, pressure, and respiration chart carefully over the next few days. Routine observation for 24–48 hours is sufficient aftercare to detect the exceptionally rare complications of bleeding or infection. Scrotal oedema has been described after paracentesis, especially when tapping of ascites is associated with laparoscopy: it responds to simple management. If several litres of fluid have been removed the patient's condition should be monitored for 24–48 hours. Initially the pulse should be recorded every half hour and blood pressure every hour. Urine output should be collected for several days, and it is wise to weigh the patient and to check the circulating levels of urea and electrolytes until the patient achieves a stable state.

In patients with malignant ascites persistent leakage through puncture wounds is sometimes a problem. For this reason incisions in the abdominal wall should be kept as small as possible and sufficient fluid removed to reduce the pressure in the abdominal cavity.

Interpretation of results

The collaboration of clinician and pathologist is important in assessing the evidence obtained from an examination of intra-abdominal fluid. Table II summarises the results to be expected, but these must be interpreted cautiously.

Fluid is removed from the peritoneal cavity most often in patients with ascites due to cirrhosis, especially when a complication is suspected. In uncomplicated cases the fluid from a patient with cirrhosis is clear and yellow, contains few white cells, and has a low concentration of total protein. A high white cell count may indicate spontaneous bacterial peritonitis; a high protein concentration may point to hepatoma; and high amylase activity is associated with pancreatic disease. Nevertheless, 10% of patients with ascites secondary to uncomplicated cirrhosis have white cell counts of over $1 \times 10^9/l$ (1000/mm^3), and high protein concentrations have been described in a similar proportion.

Table II—Guide to results of laboratory tests on ascitic fluid

Source of ascites	Appearance	Protein concentration (g/l)	Total white cell count (× 10⁹/l)	Polymorpho-nuclear leucocytes (%)	Lymphocytes (%)	Amylase activity	Microscopy	Culture
Uncomplicated cirrhosis	Clear	<30 (occasionally high)	<0·3 (occasionally high)	<25	>75	Low	Negative	Negative
Neoplasia	Bloodstained or clear	>25 (sometimes low)	0·1–1·0	<50	>50	Low	Usually positive	Negative
Pancreatitis	Clear or serosanguinous	>30	Variable	Variable	Variable	High	Negative	Negative
Tuberculosis	Clear–cloudy	>30	Variable	<50	>50	Low	Positive peritoneal biopsy	Positive
Nephrosis	Clear	<10	<0·3	<25	>75	Low	Negative	Negative
Cardiac decompensation	Clear	Variable (sometimes high)	<0·3	<25	>75	Low	Negative	Negative
Spontaneous bacterial peritonitis	Cloudy	>25	>0·3	>75	<25	Low	Often positive	Positive

Therapeutic implications

Occasionally in patients with massive ascites a large quantity of fluid may have to be removed. This may best be performed through the avascular linea alba. Anaesthetise and cleanse the abdominal wall and pass a plastic intravenous cannula (14 G) through it. Remove the introducer and thread the cannula into the abdomen until fluid flows freely. Connect the cannula to a drainage bag and control the flow of fluid with an adjustable clip. Remove up to two litres over about four hours (rapid removal of fluid may cause hypotension). If necessary reposition the patient or the cannula to maintain the flow of fluid. Cytotoxic agents may be introduced through the cannula in appropriate dosage. After sufficient fluid has been removed take out the cannula and apply a firm dressing.

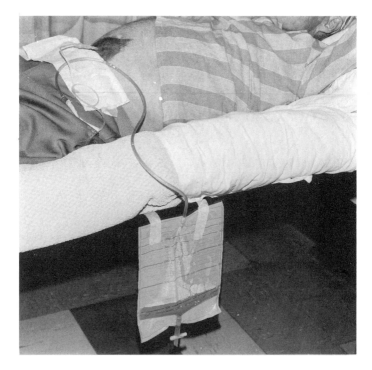

Peritoneal dialysis

E R MAHER

J R CURTIS

Indications

Peritoneal dialysis is usually performed for acute or chronic renal failure, but may also be undertaken for pulmonary oedema, removal of toxins, hypothermia, and hypercalcaemia. When faced with a patient with renal failure you must first decide whether dialysis is necessary and then, if so, whether peritoneal dialysis or haemodialysis should be performed. General guidelines for dialysis in renal failure are hyperkalaemia ($>6\cdot5$ mmol/l), acidosis (pH $<7\cdot1$), urea >40 mmol/l, or pulmonary oedema unresponsive to medical treatment. The advantages of peritoneal dialysis over haemodialysis are its relative simplicity and lack of life threatening complications. Peritoneal dialysis is preferred for patients with cardiovascular instability, for those in whom vascular access is difficult, and for those for whom anticoagulation would be hazardous.

Contraindications

Contraindications are:
- Recent abdominal surgery or trauma
- Extensive adhesions
- Ileostomy or colostomy
- Aortic vascular graft
- Inflammatory bowel disease
- Large intra-abdominal masses
- Indications for haemodialysis, such as hypoalbuminaemia or pulmonary insufficiency
- Large abdominal herniae

Most of these are relative contraindications, which increase the risk of catheter insertion or make peritoneal dialysis technically difficult.

Haemodialysis is more efficient than peritoneal dialysis and is preferred when rapid correction of electrolyte or fluid abnormalities is required. Other disadvantages of acute peritoneal dialysis are immobility; loss of protein into the dialysate; metabolic disturbances (hyperglycaemia and hyperlipidaemia); and splinting of the diaphragm, reducing basal pulmonary ventilation. Haemodialysis is likely to be preferred for the treatment of hypercatabolic and malnourished patients or those with compromised pulmonary function,

121

such as those requiring artificial ventilation. However, the ultimate choice between the two forms of dialysis is often determined by local resources and availability.

Equipment

- Sterile gown, gloves, and mask
- Sterile surgical drapes
- Skin cleaning fluid
- Local anaesthetic
- 10 ml syringe, 21, 23, and 25 G needles
- 12 gauze swabs
- 16 G intravenous cannula
- Scalpel and No 11 blade
- Scissors, skin stitch, and needle
- Catheter: Trocath stylet catheter unit (McGaw Laboratories) or silicone peritoneal dialysis catheter (single or double cuff) with guide wire, introducer, and peelaway sheath (Cook Inc)
- Peritoneal dialysis fluid (for example, 1·5% dextrose one litre bag and connecting set)
- 1 litre 0·9% NaCl and giving set

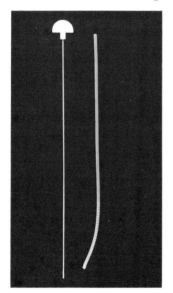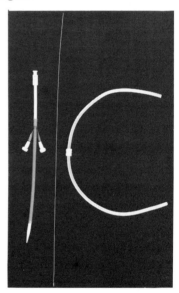

Two types of catheter: Trocath stylet catheter unit (left) and single cuff silicone peritoneal dialysis catheter with guide wire, introducer, and peelaway sheath (right).

Many instruments are contained in an intravenous cut-down pack. We shall describe two methods of catheter insertion: one with a Trocath catheter and stylet unit and the second using a guide wire method. We favour the guide wire method as it is less traumatic and the catheter can be used for long term dialysis. The choice of method will depend on the physician's experience and the availability of catheters.

Before you start

(1) Obtain the consent of the patient.

(2) Ensure that the patient's bladder is empty (usually catheterisation is necessary).

(3) Warm dialysis fluid and 1 litre of 0·9% saline to body temperature.

(4) If necessary correct coagulation abnormalities before starting.

Procedure

A General

(1) Select a site for catheter insertion and clean skin with an iodine or chlorhexidine solution. The most common sites are in the midline, one third of the way from the umbilicus to the pubic symphysis (best site for the inexperienced), and in either iliac fossa level with the anterior superior iliac spine about 2 cm lateral to the rectus sheath. Sites of surgical scars should be avoided.

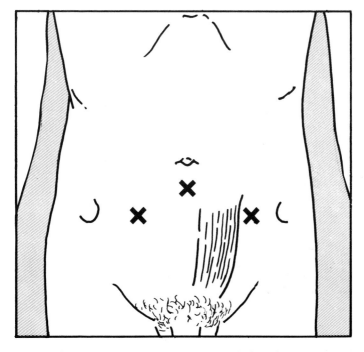

Sites for insertion of peritoneal dialysis catheters.

(2) Anaesthetise down to the peritoneum with 5 ml of 2% lignocaine.

(3) Make a small skin incision no wider than the diameter of the catheter.

(4) Ask the patient (if conscious and cooperative) to tense his abdominal musculature (for example, by lifting his head against resistance). During this manoeuvre insert a 16 G

123

intravenous cannula down to the peritoneum; there will be a slight give as you go through the peritoneum. Then advance the plastic sleeve and remove the needle. Infuse 1 litre of prewarmed 0·9% saline into the peritoneal cavity.

B   Trocath method

(1) Remove the 16 G intravenous cannula. Then remove the plastic sleeve and insert the tip of the stylet–catheter unit through the skin incision.

(2) Ask the patient to tense his abdomen again (see A(4)), and carefully push the stylet and catheter through the abdominal wall with a twisting action. As the peritoneum is punctured there is a sudden decrease in resistance. Excessive entry of the stylet may be prevented by holding the lower end of the stylet–catheter unit just above the skin.

(3) On entering the peritoneal cavity, the stylet should be withdrawn 2–3 cm and the stylet and catheter advanced downwards into the pelvis at about 60° to the skin until about two thirds of the catheter has been inserted. The final part of the catheter is then advanced, as the stylet is withdrawn, until about 2 cm of catheter is left above the skin. The end of the catheter can then be attached to the connecting set to check that dialysis fluid will run in freely. If it does not withdraw the catheter slightly and try again.

(4) Put a purse string suture around the catheter to prevent leakage, but do not overtighten.

(5) Secure the catheter by pushing the metal disc over the catheter so that it lies against a gauze swab on the skin surface. Be careful not to bend the disc as then it will not retain the catheter. Trim the catheter so that 2 cm lie above the skin, and then reattach the connecting set. The L shaped connector should be supported in position by a wad of gauze to prevent kinking.

C   Guide wire method

(1) Follow general steps A(1) to A(4).

(2) Insert a 0·038 in guide wire through the intravenous cannula into the peritoneal cavity, then remove the intravenous cannula. Use blunt dissection to make a small subcutaneous pocket for the dacron cuff on the catheter.

(3) Thread the introducer and peelaway sheath unit over the guide wire. Then ask the patient to tense his abdomen; push the introducer and sheath into the peritoneal cavity and direct it towards the pelvis. When the peelaway sheath is in position, withdraw the introducer and guide wire.

(4) A single cuff soft silicone peritoneal dialysis catheter is then threaded through the sheath up to the level of the dacron cuff. The outer sheath is then peeled away and the catheter advanced so that the cuff lies subcutaneously. A purse string suture can be inserted as necessary.

(5) In patients likely to need long term peritoneal dialysis, a

double cuff Tenckhoff catheter can be inserted as above, except that a portion of the catheter is tunnelled so that the second cuff lies subcutaneously.

(6) The catheter can then be attached to the peritoneal dialysis connecting line.

Problems

Failure to drain may be due to a variety of causes. First, check the tubing is not kinked. If the catheter is blocked by fibrin flushing with heparin or urokinase may improve the flow. Treating constipation or changing the patient's position can also improve catheter function. If the catheter has been inserted into the preperitoneal space then failure to drain will be associated with swelling or oedema of the abdomen or scrotum. If the catheter is displaced from the pelvis or encased by omentum then the catheter must be repositioned or replaced.

Dialysate leakage may be controlled by a purse string around the catheter or reducing the exchange volume.

Blood in dialysate usually clears after a few exchanges. Heparin (250 U/l) may be added to the dialysate to prevent clots blocking the catheter.

Complications

Bowel perforation is recognised by the presence of faecal material in the dialysate or the onset of dextrostix positive watery diarrhoea. The catheter should be removed, antibiotics started—for example, metronidazole, cefuroxime, tobramycin—and a surgical opinion on laparatomy sought.

Peritonitis is usually caused by contamination during bag changes and so should be prevented by careful technique. It presents with cloudy bags and abdominal pain. Microscopy of the dialysate shows white cells and organisms. Intraperitoneal antibiotics (cefuroxime 200 mg/l and tobramycin 6 mg/l) are commenced until culture and sensitivities are available. Pain may be ameliorated by adding 10 ml of 1% lignocaine to the dialysate.

Aftercare

Peritoneal dialysis is commonly started with hourly 1 litre exchanges (10 minutes inflow, 30 minutes dwell, and 20 minutes outflow). If fluid removal is required every third or second exchange may be performed with a hypertonic bag (4·5% dextrose). Plasma potassium should be checked and potassium added to the dialysate bags as necessary. Hyperglycaemia may also occur, particularly if 4·5% dialysate is

125

used. Trocath catheters should be replaced after 48 hours, but single or double cuff silicone catheters can be used for long term dialysis.

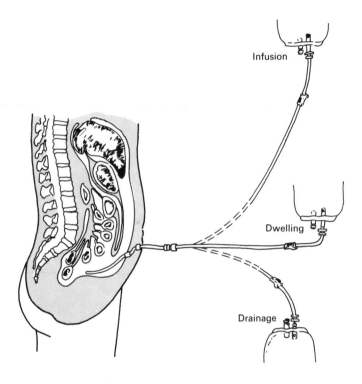

Technique of peritoneal dialysis.

Lumbar puncture

J M S PEARCE

Indications

Lumbar puncture should not be indulged in idly as a result of diagnostic bankruptcy nor in place of a neurological opinion. Though it may be informative in certain patients with coma or stroke it should not be done blindly as an immediate procedure until other diagnostic tests have been performed.

There are three main indications: (a) for diagnostic purposes (see table); (b) for introducing contrast media; and (c) for introducing chemotherapeutic agents—for example, in meningitis or leukaemia.

Indications for performing lumbar puncture for diagnosis	Tests
Suspected subarachnoid haemorrhage	Blood, xanthochromia
Selected strokes, but not routinely	Red blood cells, protein
Myelopathies and suspected multiple sclerosis (but not for suspected cord compression)	Protein, IgG, or gammaglobulin Oligoclonal bands
Peripheral neuropathies—for example, Guillain–Barré syndrome	Cells, protein
Infections of central nervous system (bacterial meningitis; tuberculosis; acute and subacute encephalitides; neurosyphilis; viral, fungal, and protozoal meningitis)	Cells, protein, treponemal haemagglutinating antibody (or other specific tests), glucose, culture, virology, special stains and antibodies

Contraindications

These are:
(1) Raised intracranial pressure, indicated by morning or postural headache, vomiting, and papilloedema. Even in the absence of signs, a history suspicious of increased pressure contraindicates lumbar puncture and should lead to a neurological consultation and CT scan. The danger is of fatal transtentorial or cerebellar "coning."
(2) Suspected cord compression. In many isolated cord lesions it is not possible to distinguish an intrinsic lesion (for example, multiple sclerosis) from extrinsic compression by disc or tumour. Diagnostic lumbar puncture does not resolve this problem. Myelography with simulta-

neous cerebrospinal fluid examination and/or a spinal CT scan are the investigations of choice.

(3) Local sepsis. Puncture through infected skin carries the risk of meningitis; lumbar puncture must be avoided.

Procedure

The most important factor in achieving an easy lumbar puncture is the correct positioning of the patient. The procedure should be explained to the patient and he should be comfortable and relaxed.

Place the patient on his left side with his back right up against the edge of the bed or firm trolley. Both legs are flexed towards the chest: place a pillow between the legs to ensure that the back is vertical. The neck should be slightly flexed.

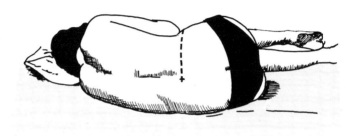

Mask and gloves should be worn. Clean the skin with iodine and spirit (or other antiseptic) and then position the sterile drapes. Use a 22 to 25 small gauge needle if possible to avoid a larger hole in the dura; but in a rigid "arthritic spine" a larger, 18 to 20 G needle will sometimes prove necessary. When using the needle try to keep the bevel in the vertical, axial plane of the dural fibres, thus minimising the size of the hole.

Palpate the anterior–superior iliac spine. The interspace perpendicularly beneath it is that at L3–4. Since the spinal cord ends at L1–2 the spaces above and below L3–4 are equally acceptable sites. Palpate the spinous processes superior to the chosen interspace: the needle will be inserted about 1 cm inferior to the tip of the process.

Draw up 5 ml of lignocaine 2% plain and, stretching the skin evenly over the interspace, infiltrate the skin and deeper tissues.

Allow at least one minute for the lignocaine to work then introduce the needle. Make sure that the needle is 90° to the back, with its bevel in the sagittal plane and pointing slightly to the head. Push the needle through the resistance of the superficial supraspinous ligament. The interspinous ligament is then easily negotiated. At about 4–7 cm the firmer resistance of the ligamentum flavum is felt, when an extra push will result in a popping sensation as the dura is breached.

The needle should now lie in the subarachnoid space, and when the stylet is withdrawn clear colourless fluid should drip out.

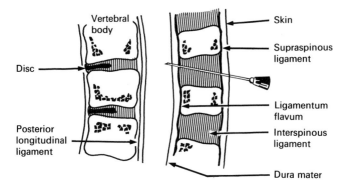

Dry tap

If no fluid emerges or it does not flow easily rotate the needle, because a flap of dura may be lying against the bevel. If there is still no fluid reinsert the stylet and cautiously advance, withdrawing the stylet after each movement. Pain radiating down either leg indicates that the needle is too lateral and has hit nerve roots. Withdraw the needle almost completely, check the patient's position, and reinsert in the midline.

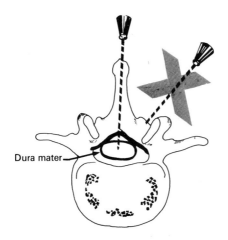

If the needle meets total obstruction do not force it as the needle may be lying against an intervertebral disc and could damage it. Again, withdraw the needle, check its position, and reinsert. If there is complete failure move one space up or down depending on the original position. The procedure may be easier if the patient is sitting up.

A dry tap is usually due to a failure of technique. After two or three attempts a colleague should be invited to show his superior skill. Rare causes of a genuine dry tap are arachnoiditis and infiltrations of the meninges.

129

Manometry

When the cerebrospinal fluid (CSF) flows freely the pressure should be measured. A manometer is connected to the hub of the needle directly or through a two way tap. An assistant holds the top end and pressure is recorded (normal 80–180 mm CSF). The height of the meniscus should be seen to change with respiration. Pressure on the jugular veins should cause a rise of > 40 mm pressure (a negative Queckenstedt's test), but this should no longer be used in place of myelography if obstruction of the spinal canal is suspected.

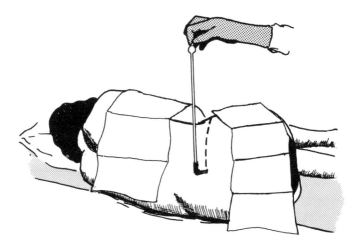

Spinal block causes a failure of free rise and fall (positive Queckenstedt) and is usually accompanied by yellowish CSF with a high protein content (Froin's syndrome).

The commonest cause of low CSF pressure is bad needle placement, but if the low pressure is genuine no attempt should be made to aspirate as the cause may be obstruction of CSF flow caused by cerebellar tonsil herniation or spinal block. In either case a neurological opinion is needed.

A slightly raised CSF pressure in a very anxious or fat patient may be ignored. Pressures over 250 mm are abnormal and should be investigated. If a greatly raised pressure is discovered in a clear fluid the CSF should be collected from the manometer and the needle withdrawn. The patient should be nursed flat and a neurologist or neurosurgeon consulted.

Specimens for diagnosis

Eight to 10 ml of CSF are collected. The minimal requirements are a record of opening pressure, total and differential cell count, and total protein. There are no other routine tests and additional studies are dictated by the clinical queries and by close liaison with the local laboratories. Glucose is unnecessary unless an infective or neoplastic meningitis is considered; Lange curves, Pandy tests, and chlorides are obsolete.

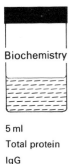

Biochemistry	Microbiology	Ward
5 ml	2 ml	1 ml
Total protein	Cells and differential	? xanthochromia
IgG	Gram stain	
Oligoclonal bands	Culture	
Glucose	Special stains for fungi, cryptococci, TB	
	Viral agglutinins, millipore for malignant cells	
	VDRL and TPHA	

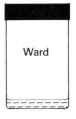

A ward specimen of 1 ml is useful in suspected subarachnoid bleeding, in which xanthochromia (a yellow discoloured supernatant) may be observed before the laboratory report. It may also be a useful spare for "mislaid specimens."

Even the most careful lumbar puncture can be bedevilled by bloodstaining. Bloody fluid should be collected in three tubes. A traumatic tap can be distinguished from subarachnoid haemorrhage in three ways.

Firstly, blood due to trauma forms streams in an otherwise clear CSF, while the CSF of subarachnoid bleeding is diffusely bloodstained.

Secondly, on centrifugation or standing the supernatant is colourless in a traumatic tap but xanthochromic in subarachnoid haemorrhage. The only exception is that a clear supernatant may rarely occur if the lumbar puncture is done within six hours of a subarachnoid haemorrhage occurring.

Thirdly, the first three consecutive specimens of CSF in a traumatic tap show clearing of the blood and usually become colourless, with a corresponding fall of the red cell count.

Aftercare and complications

Once the specimens have been collected the needle is removed. The patient may be nursed flat, prone or tilted head down for 24 hours, but it is debatable whether this hallowed routine lessens the incidence of headache. Headache after lumbar puncture is a low intracranial pressure state due to persistent leakage of CSF through the hole(s) in the dura. Prevention demands a careful technique and the use of a small gauge needle. Headache occurs in about 10% of patients and may be accompanied by vomiting. It is treated by laying the patient flat, bed tilted head down, and by the liberal use of analgesics (aspirin, paracetamol, or codeine phosphate) with antiemetics (metaclopramide or domperidone). It usually lasts 36 to 72 hours, but may occasionally persist for a week. The onset may be delayed for three or four days. A similar picture occurs after spinal anaesthetic; many anaesthetists use an "epidural blood patch" to prevent or to treat this condition.

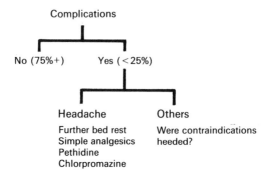

Complications

No (75%+)   Yes (<25%)

Headache
Further bed rest
Simple analgesics
Pethidine
Chlorpromazine

Others
Were contraindications heeded?

Interpretation of results

CSF: some normal values

		Diagnostic value
Opening pressure	50–180 mm CSF	Raised intracranial pressure
Osmolarity	295 mosmol/l*	Rarely
pH	7·31*	Rarely
Total WBCs	0–5/mm³	Inflammatory states
Total protein	0·15–0·45 g/l	Non-specific
Gamma globulin	3–12% of total	(immune or demyelinating
IgG	<0·06 g/l	diseases)
Glucose	2–4·5 mmol/l	Pyogenic, fungal, TB, malignant infiltrations
VDRL, TPHA, TPI	Negative	Syphilis
Lactate	1·6 mmol/l*	Pyogenic meningitis
Ammonia	300 μg/l*	Hepatic encephalopathy Reye's syndrome

*Average values.

CSF findings should always be interpreted in the light of clinical features and other laboratory results. A raised CSF protein always implies a lesion of the CNS but is itself seldom diagnostic.

Some CSF profiles

Purulent: high WBC, mainly polymorphs, low glucose ±

Infections
    Bacterial meningitis, viral meningitis (early)
    TB meningitis (early)
    Cerebral abscess, subdural empyema, intracranial thrombophlebitis

Non-infectious
    Chemical meningitis (for example, after contrast media)
    Mollaret's recurrent meningitis

Lymphocytic: high WBC, mainly lymphocytes, low glucose

Infections
    TB, fungal, treponemal, leptospiral, listeria and half treated bacterial
      meningitis
    Viral meningitis

Non-infectious
    Carcinomatous, lymphomatous, leukaemic "meningitis"
    Sarcoidosis

Lymphocytic: high WBC, mainly lymphocytes, normal glucose

Infections
    Viral meningitis, encephalitis (for example, herpes simplex)
    Half treated bacterial meningitis
    Parameningeal infections (abscess, intracranial thrombophlebitis)
    Fungal and TB meningitis (early)
    Parasitic infestation (for example, trichinosis, toxoplasmosis,
      amoebiasis)

Non-infectious
    Post-infectious encephalitis, myelitis
    Acute demyelination (MS)

Proctoscopy and sigmoidoscopy

D J ELLIS

Introduction

Both proctoscopy and sigmoidoscopy are used for diagnosis, treatment, and follow up. Lesions of the anal canal, rectum, and lower sigmoid colon can be diagnosed and biopsy carried out. Rectal swabs are sent for bacteriological studies or specimens of faeces for identification of parasites. Internal haemorrhoids can be treated by injection, rubber band ligation, or cryotherapy through a proctoscope. Excision or diathermy of small localised lesions and deflations of a sigmoid volvulus may be carried out through a sigmoidoscope. Follow up examinations are useful to monitor progress of disease—for example, improvement in non-specific proctitis after a course of steroid enemas and for the detection of recurrent malignancy.

Indications

Proctoscopy or sigmoidoscopy, or both, should be carried out on all patients who complain of the following symptoms or signs:
- piles
- rectal bleeding
- change of bowel habit, especially recurring attacks of diarrhoea
- pain or difficulty in defaecation
- lesions around the anal opening (abscesses, fistulae, discharge, ulcers, external piles, pruritus)
- prolapse.

Contraindications

Painful digital examination requires further investigation under general anaesthesia. Sigmoidoscopy should be undertaken with care in patients with suspected toxic dilatation of the colon.

Preparation

Pre-examination bowel preparation is generally unnecessary and may disguise abnormalities by producing oedema of the rectal and colonic mucosa. It may, however, be necessary in patients with heavy faecal loading of the distal colon and rectum. A Microlax or phosphate enema is usually necessary prior to fibreoptic flexible sigmoidoscopy.

Equipment

The following must be available:
- Examination gloves
- Lubricating jelly
- Anglepoise lamp and light source with the right connections
- Cotton wool pledgets with holder
- Incowipes
- Proctoscope
- Sigmoidoscope with insufflation bulb (the plastic disposable type are to be preferred for better illumination)
- Biopsy forceps
- Sucker of some kind (preferably guarded)
- Container for biopsy specimens

More specialised equipment will be mentioned under Procedure.

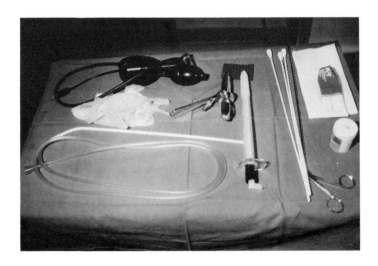

Procedure

Proctoscopy

Proctoscopy can be done without difficulty or discomfort in the doctor's surgery or outpatient clinic without general anaesthesia. It is important to ensure that the patient is lying in the correct position and is comfortable and relaxed. The left lateral position is usually advocated, with the buttocks pushed backwards and both hips flexed, the right leg above the left to tilt the anal opening upwards. In obese patients it is helpful to place a cushion under the buttocks.

135

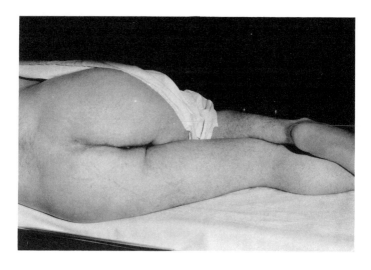

The first step is to separate the buttocks and inspect the anal verge carefully for pruritus, external piles, a fissure, or a fistula. It is essential to insert the lubricated forefinger (fingernail uppermost) through the anal canal and examine the anal canal and lower part of the rectum before attempting to pass a proctoscope or sigmoidoscope. If there is anal stenosis or severe pain further examination should be under general anaesthesia.

The calibre of the anal canal should be judged at the preliminary examination with the index finger, and too large an instrument should not be used. Assuming the equipment required is available and working, the proctoscope should first be warmed under the hot tap, dried, and lubricated. It is passed by pushing the head of the obturator firmly but gently through the anal canal in the direction of the umbilicus, and when through the anus it is turned in the direction of the patient's head and inserted to the hilt. The obturator must be kept fully engaged in the proctoscope during insertion to avoid nipping the anal mucosa. Close inspection is made as the instrument is withdrawn, firstly of the lower rectal mucosa and then of the anal canal. Make note of any haemorrhoids, internal fistulous openings, and the linear raw area of a fissure. Observation of the bowel contents and mucosa is described later under Sigmoidoscopy.

Injecting internal haemorrhoids—An injecting proctoscope is used for this procedure and rotated so as to allow the pile to bulge in the side aperture. Through a special haemorrhoid needle 3–5 ml of 5% phenol in oil is injected submucosally into the base of the pile; the injection must not be intravascular. This procedure should be painless; if not suspect the injection is in the wrong place.

Rubber band ligation—Using either grasping forceps or suction the pile is pulled into the collar of the ligation gun and two rubber bands placed around the "neck" of the pile. It is important that the pile is grasped proximal to its main bulge and above the dentate line. If done lower the patient will experience pain.

136

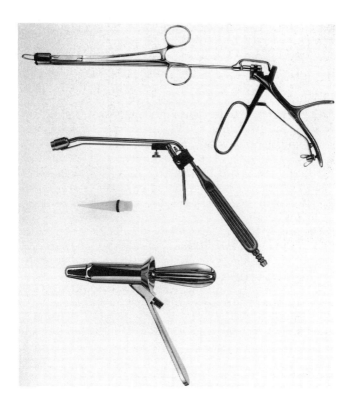

Sigmoidoscopy

This can usually be done in the outpatient clinic without anaesthesia, when again the left lateral position is to be preferred. Sometimes it is difficult to advance the sigmoidoscope beyond the rectosigmoid junction (15 cm) owing to discomfort or lack of experience. In this situation the procedure is best undertaken under general anaesthesia and in the lithotomy position with head down tilt on the table. Occasionally the knee–elbow position may allow full inspection without general anaesthesia. Procedures through the operating sigmoidoscope are also preferred to be done in the lithotomy position under general or local anaesthesia.

Before sigmoidoscopy the lower abdomen should first be palpated for the presence of a mass; digital palpation of the rectum then follows and finally bimanual palpation with the right index finger in the rectum and the left hand on the lower abdomen.

The sigmoidoscope is introduced in a similar way to the proctoscope, but as soon as the end has penetrated the anal canal the obturator is removed. The illuminated eyepiece with insufflating bulb is attached. The insufflating bulb is an important part of the instrument as the upper half of the rectum and lower sigmoid can be seen clearly only when air is blown in to distend the lumen. The instrument is advanced under visual control and the rectal mucosa examined carefully from below upwards. When the upper rectum is reached the end of the sigmoidoscope is moved to the patient's left backwards, and then forwards to round the rectosigmoid bend into the lower sigmoid colon. It is vital to get a clear view of this area, as it cannot be felt digitally from the rectum or by lower abdominal palpation. The operator must be prepared patiently to clear the rectum of faeces by digital removal, scooping them out in the sigmoidoscope or using pledgets on forceps that have long handles. A sucker must always be available but used gently and its end guarded with a rubber tube. The sigmoidoscope must never be forced upwards, and blanching of the mucosa is a danger sign.

The mucous membrane is inspected for colour, texture, and mobility. Inflammation, erosions, ulcers, adenomas, polyps, and the raised or ulcerated edge of a carcinoma are looked for. Areas of inflammation or erosions are biopsied, preferably with the newer "mucosa only" forceps and preferably below about 8 cm. High anterior biopsies run the risk of perforation. Polyps and carcinomas can be biopsied with the larger bite alligator forceps and multiple specimens should be taken. Vascular lesions should be biopsied with care or not at all. The barrel of the sigmoidoscope is calibrated in centimetres, and the distance of any lesion from the anal verge must be noted. The presence of blood, mucus, or pus in the lumen should be noted and also the colour, consistency, and shape of the faecal masses—for example, diverticular disease can be diagnosed by finding a contracted, corrugated faecal cast.

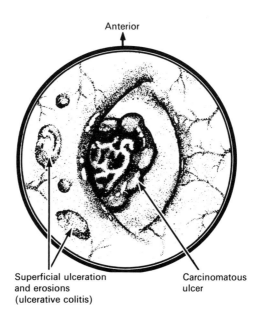

Anterior

Superficial ulceration and erosions (ulcerative colitis)

Carcinomatous ulcer

Proctoscopy should be done after sigmoidoscopy as anal lesions may be missed through the sigmoidoscope.

Flexible sigmoidoscopy—The fibreoptic flexible sigmoidoscope is increasing in use as it allows visualisation of much more of the colon. However, its use requires familiarity with the use of fibreoptic endoscopic equipment.

The use of the operating sigmoidoscope for diathermy excision etc is beyond the scope of this chapter.

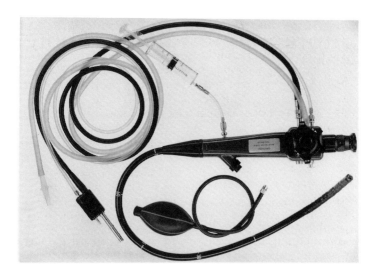

Troubleshooting

Perforation of the bowel should be recognised and assessment made regarding laparotomy. Bleeding may sometimes be a problem but is usually controlled by gentle pressure through the sigmoidoscope. Heavy bleeding may be controlled by packing of the rectum or suture and observation of the patient in hospital; note that blood may pass proximally in the bowel and not be immediately apparent.

Specimens

Specimens should be accurately labelled and sufficient clinical details given to the pathologist. All findings must be noted carefully, and are best presented in diagrammatic form.

Suprapubic catheterisation

PAUL HILTON

Introduction

Catheterisation of the bladder is one of the most commonly performed surgical procedures, and is currently used in up to 20% of all patients in hospital; it should, however, never be undertaken lightly, since it carries a significant morbidity and mortality. It is the commonest cause of nosocomially acquired infection, accounting for 35% of such events; approximately 1% of infected cases may become bacteraemic, and in these there is a threefold increase in mortality. For the remainder catheterisation may mean considerable discomfort, an increased stay in hospital, and financial implications for the health service. Cystotomy, the creation of an artificial opening into the bladder, is most often performed suprapubically and may circumvent many of the problems associated with urethral catheterisation. There is little information on the relative use made of different catheterisation techniques, but a recent survey of practices among gynaecologists in the United Kingdom showed that less than 40% favoured the suprapubic approach for postoperative bladder drainage, although of those with a major interest in urology over 60% advocated this route. The procedure may be performed either by an open operation or by a closed stab procedure, and either may be carried out in the ward under local anaesthesia, or in the operating theatre under general or regional anaesthesia. Although most of the following comments relate to closed suprapubic stab cystotomy, the same general principles of insertion technique and aftercare apply in all cases.

Indications

Acute urinary retention

Pain from acute urinary retention should be relieved as quickly as possible, and if simple measures to promote voiding are not successful catheterisation must be undertaken. In men the passage of a urethral catheter is often painful, and if the first attempt is unsuccessful repeated attempts may lead to the formation of a false passage, infection, and stricture. In women these problems are uncommon, but nevertheless retention is often treated by repeated urethral catheterisation when a single suprapubic catheterisation would suffice.

Chronic urinary retention

The finding of a significant residual urine volume in the bladder is not in itself an indication for drainage; however, the development of recurrent or persistent urinary infection, evidence of upper tract deterioration, or of chronic retention with "overflow" incontinence may necessitate catheterisation. Long term suprapubic drainage may be the most appropriate in some circumstances.

Postoperative use

All gynaecological, urological, and rectal surgery may be associated with postoperative urinary retention as a result of pain, distortion of local anatomy, clot retention, pelvic haematoma or periurethral oedema, or by virtue of bladder denervation or neuropraxia. Catheterisation may therefore be necessary following any such procedure, and is perhaps best used prophylactically in many situations. The advantage of a suprapubic catheter is that the patient's ability to void can be assessed without removing the catheter. This appreciably reduces patient discomfort, nursing time, and urinary infection, since repeated catheterisations become unnecessary.

Urethral trauma, urethral or bladder neck surgery, and repair of vesical or urethral fistula

Catheterisation is positively indicated in these situations to allow healing of a suture line in the bladder or urethra and to prevent the development of, or promote the healing of, a urinary fistula. Urethral catheterisation may not only further damage the mucosa but also encourage local oedema and delay healing.

Acute vulvovaginitis

Acute vulval or vaginal inflammatory conditions, particularly those associated with herpetic infection, may necessitate suprapubic catheterisation.

Intractable urinary incontinence

Rarely, catheterisation may be required for the management of urinary incontinence which is unresponsive to alternative methods of treatment and where pads and collection devices do not render a socially acceptable level of continence. As with chronic retention with overflow, long term suprapubic drainage may be the most appropriate in some circumstances.

Contraindications

Inability to distend the bladder

Ideally the bladder should be distended with 500 ml, though with experience 300 ml may be adequate. At lower volumes the danger of perforating the bowel becomes too great to justify the closed procedure.

141

Gross haematuria or clot retention

The fine calibre of most catheters designed for closed suprapubic insertion (6–16 FG) makes them unsuitable for use in the presence of gross haematuria; a larger catheter (22 FG) inserted by open cystotomy is more appropriate where there is a risk of occlusion by clot.

Known or suspected carcinoma of the bladder

The risk of implanting malignant cells into a fistulous track makes even suspected carcinoma an absolute contraindication.

Recent cystotomy

An open technique at the time of operation is preferable to closed catheterisation, as this may disrupt the vesical suture line.

Equipment

Before catheterisation all materials necessary for the procedure should be to hand. A prepacked "catheterisation tray" is useful, but otherwise the following materials should be assembled.

Postoperative insertion: bladder undistended
- Antiseptic solution for urethral preparation (for example, chlorhexidine 0.25%)
- Non-retaining urethral catheter (for example, Nelaton, 12–14 FG)
- Infusion set with 500 ml irrigating fluid

Insertion under local anaesthetic
- Local anaesthetic (for example, 5–10 ml, 1–2% lignocaine)
- Syringe and needles
- Sterile hand towel and gloves
- Galley pots and receiver

All cases
- Antiseptic solution for skin preparation (for example, providone iodine)
- No 11 scalpel blade
- Sterile swabs or cotton wool balls
- 00 silk suture
- Urine drainage bag
- Adhesive tape

Choice of catheter

A Foley or Malecot catheter may be inserted suprapubically either by cutting down onto a sound or by means of the Robertson cystotrocar. Both methods are simple and straightforward, although more usually one of the several catheter types specifically designed for closed suprapubic insertion is used. The following are among those currently in use.

Bonanno catheter (Becton–Dickinson Ltd) — This is a very fine catheter (6 FG) with an inner insertion trocar which therefore has the advantage of a minimal insertion force; it is, however, for the same reason, not suitable for situations where urine is heavily bloodstained. The distal end of the catheter has a preformed pigtail memory curve which prevents its passage through the urethra. Drainage is via an end hole and several side holes placed around the inside of the curve to avoid occlusion by the bladder mucosa. There is a concertina support to allow bending of the catheter at the skin surface without kinking and a small ovoid flange which is sutured to the skin; this allows the catheter to be inserted close to a suprapubic incision and to remain in place for three to four weeks. It is therefore ideally suited to postoperative use.

Stamey percutaneous catheter (Cook Inc) — This is a curved polyethylene catheter available in 10, 12, and 14 FG. It is secured in the bladder by a flange of the Malecot type and its curved shape allows easy taping to the abdominal wall. Because of the shape and width of the catheter tip in relation to the insertion needle a relatively high insertion force is required, with a consequent risk of damage to the posterior bladder wall.

Cystofix (B Braun Ltd) — This is a polyurethane catheter of 10 or 15 FG. It has a memory curve like the Bonanno catheter, but is passed through the inside of the trocar, in contrast to most other catheters described; the trocars themselves are of 12 and 17 FG respectively, and although their shape ensures insertion with minimal force they involve a risk of extensive tissue "coring." The catheters are sutured to the skin with the aid of a grooved supporting flange.

Cystocath (Dow Corning Corporation) — This is a soft, 8 or 12 FG silicone elastomer catheter. It has a separate insertion trocar and cannula; once this device is in the bladder the inner trocar is removed and the catheter passed through the cannula. The conical shape of the 8 FG trocar necessitates a higher insertion force than the Bonanno, and the "two stage" insertion leads to a rather messy procedure, with considerable urine leakage. The catheter is secured in place with a silastic disc of 7·5 cm diameter fixed with a medical grade adhesive; this limits the functional life of the catheter, and makes attachment close to a suprapubic incision problematic. The soft catheter material causes little local irritation and is generally comfortable in use. One particular problem of this construction is that the catheter is readily passed per urethram once voiding is initiated; although the problem is easily overcome by withdrawing the device suprapubically until it returns to the bladder, this is associated with a risk of infection. The Cystocath is perhaps most useful for bladder drainage after vaginal surgery.

Simplastic (Franklin Medical) — This catheter is made of polyvinylchloride and is available in 10, 12, and 16 FG and is inserted using an inner insertion trocar. It is retained in the bladder by a balloon on the shaft and a locking flange on the

143

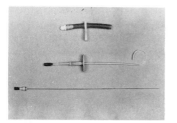

Bonanno.

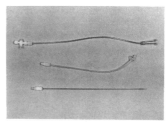

Stamey.

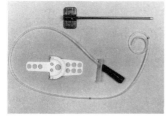

Cystofix.

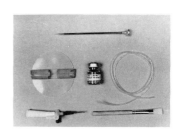

Cystocath.

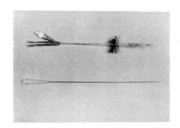

Simplastic.

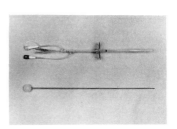

Ingram.

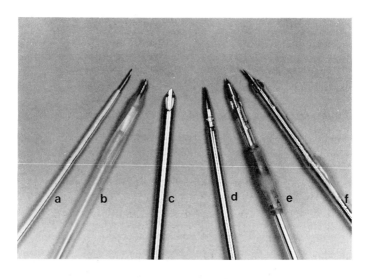

Catheter tips: (a) Bonanno; (b) Stamey; (c) Cystofix; (d) Cystocath; (e) Simplastic; (f) Ingram.

skin surface. The balloon on this and the Argyle catheter may cause difficulties in insertion unless a generous skin and sheath incision is made. The rigid construction means that suction can be applied without collapse, and the negative electrostatic charge associated with the plastic is said to resist encrustation and adhesion of clot.

Argyle Ingram trocar catheter (Sherwood Medical) — Similar in many respects to the Simplastic catheter the Ingram is also of plastic construction, available in 12 and 16 FG, and retained by a balloon and moveable surface flange. Being similar in tip shape to the Stamey catheter, it too suffers from the problem of requiring a high insertion force, with the risks noted above. It is generally of a more solid construction than other catheters and is unique in having a separate irrigation channel; it may therefore be useful in patients with infected urine or with heavy haematuria, although it tends to be uncomfortable for mobile patients.

Before you start

Anaesthesia

For postoperative bladder drainage the catheter is inserted under general or regional anaesthesia; otherwise local infiltration is perfectly satisfactory.

Bladder distension

When the catheter is to be used postoperatively the bladder must first be filled. Using standard aseptic techniques, a urethral catheter is passed and 400–500 ml sterile saline instilled via the infusion set.

Instructions

Insertion techniques vary considerably with different catheter designs, and the manufacturer's instructions should be studied beforehand by the operator and nursing staff. The technique described and illustrated is for the insertion of the Bonanno catheter.

Procedure

The suprapubic area is cleansed, the point of insertion being in the midline 3 cm above the pubic symphysis. In obese patients the catheter is most easily inserted in the suprapubic crease. When local anaesthesia is used the point of insertion should be infiltrated down to the bladder with 1–2% lignocaine; urine may be aspirated into the syringe to confirm correct angulation of puncture. A small stab incision made in the skin with a No 11 scalpel blade facilitates catheter introduction. The catheter or trocar, assembled according to the manufacturer's instructions, is introduced through the incision with a firm thrust in a slightly caudal direction. Resistance should be minimal once the bladder is entered, and correct siting is confirmed by the free flow of urine when the catheter is aspirated, or the trocar disengaged.

The catheter is advanced over the trocar until its flange is flat against the skin, and then the trocar is removed. The catheter is secured by suture, adhesive, balloon inflation, or tape, as appropriate, and is connected to the drainage bag which should also be secured to the skin to prevent dragging. The bladder is drained and the urethral catheter removed.

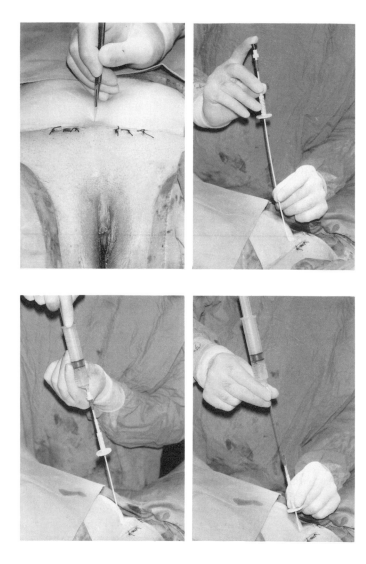

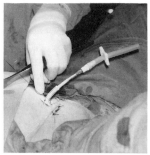

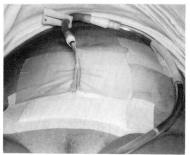

In catheters without a fixed flange or balloon (for example, Cystocath and Cystofix) or those with drainage holes proximal to their fixation (for example, Stamey) it is important to ensure that all drainage holes, and not simply the trocar tip, are advanced well into the bladder. Otherwise, as the bladder empties, the catheter may come to lie in the retropubic space, and although initial drainage may appear satisfactory failure may be recognised on return to the ward.

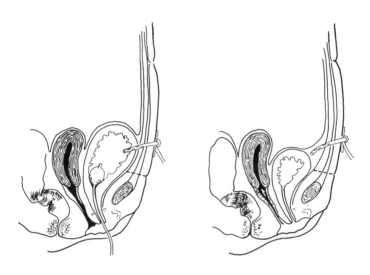

Aftercare

The catheter should be left on continuous drainage until the patient is to attempt voiding; timing will depend on the indication for catheterisation, but for postoperative drainage following incontinence surgery my preference is for three days' free drainage. The adaptor or drainage connection should be clamped, or the connecting three way tap closed first thing in the morning; on no account should the catheter itself be clamped as this will encourage fracture. If the patient cannot void, or becomes distressed, the clamp should be released to avoid overdistension of the bladder. If she achieves normal voiding the residual volume should be checked after eight hours. The habit of checking the residual volume after each void is not recommended as this may give a false impression of the efficiency of micturition by masking an accumulating residual volume. The residual volume is checked by emptying the drainage bag, allowing the patient to void when she wants to and then unclamping the catheter for five to 15 minutes (depending on catheter calibre). Although a high fluid intake may be encouraged while the catheter is on free drainage, this is to be avoided once the patient begins to attempt voiding. It will complicate the measurement of residual volumes (since the drainage will consist of the residual plus newly excreted urine), but more importantly will compromise detrusor contraction if muscle fibres are persistently overstretched by the high output.

Practices vary considerably as to what constitutes an acceptable residual volume, but it is my practice to leave the catheter on free drainage overnight until the patient achieves an evening residual volume of less than 100 ml and is voiding volumes of over 200 ml. At this stage the catheter is clamped overnight and the residual volume checked after voiding in the morning. If this, too, is less than 100 ml the catheter is then left clamped for a full 24 hours and a further residual volume checked the following morning; if this is less than 100 ml the catheter is removed. If prophylactic chemotherapy is not used—and it is not my practice to do so—urine samples should be obtained every 48 hours for culture and sensitivity testing.

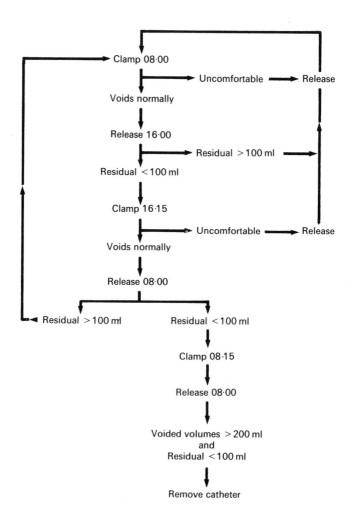

Complications

Failure to enter the bladder is rarely a problem if the bladder is adequately distended beforehand. If free flow of urine is not observed when the catheter and stylet are disengaged the catheter should be aspirated with a syringe; if urine is not obtained the whole assembly should be removed and resited after further filling. On no account must an inner trocar be advanced back into its catheter, nor should an external trocar catheter be withdrawn through its trocar; in either case perforation or fracture of the catheter may result.

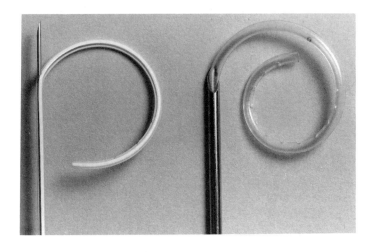

Bowel perforation is also most usually an indication of inadequate bladder filling. The catheter should be removed and resited and antibiotic therapy instituted with metronidazole and a cephalosporin. With small calibre catheters (6–8 FG) this is usually all that is necessary, although vital signs should be closely observed and evidence of peritonism sought; with any of the larger instruments laparotomy and bowel repair should be considered essential.

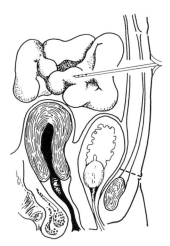

Haematuria may occur on the first day after insertion as a result of trauma caused by catheterisation, or at a later stage, through cystitis or mucosal irritation. A catheter specimen should be cultured, but in the absence of infection haematuria usually settles spontaneously.

Detachment from the skin is rarely a problem within the usual time scale of postoperative bladder drainage; it can usually be managed by resuturing or taping.

Failure of drainage may occur at any stage and usually reflects obstruction or kinking of the catheter or drainage system; dressings and taping should be checked and adjusted as necessary, and the catheter should be gently flushed with sterile saline to exclude encrustation or obstruction by clot. If no drainage results it is possible that the catheter has been extruded into the retropubic space (see Procedure); in the latter situation replacement is required.

Leakage around the catheter is much less of a problem with suprapubic than with urethral catheters, but it may arise for similar reasons to drainage failure. In the absence of these problems leakage around the catheter may result from uninhibited bladder contractions and can be treated with anticholinergic drugs. It should be borne in mind, however, that this is much less likely with a suprapubic than with a urethral catheter, and the possibility of fracture of the catheter should be considered. This is more likely with the more rigid catheters, and in particular has been reported with the original version of the Bonanno catheter; if this problem is suspected the catheter should be removed and a replacement introduced. All catheters should be checked on removal; if doubt over completeness exists radiological confirmation, and if necessary cystoscopic retrieval, should be performed.

Urethral catheterisation

C G FOWLER

Introduction

If venepuncture is the commonest form of assault in hospitals urethral catheterisation must surely be the most frequent cause of bodily harm inflicted outside the operating theatre. Bad catheterisation causes strictures in the male urethra, and a stricture can blight a man's life for years. Patience, gentleness, and a readiness to ask for help are the marks of good catheterisation.

Indications

Temporary catheterisation

Urethral catheterisation is most obviously indicated as an emergency measure to relieve the pain of acute retention. This is commonest in men with prostatic disease and bladder outflow obstruction but it can also be due to clotting of blood in the bladder, urethral stricture, or the failure of sphincter relaxation associated with postoperative pain. The female bladder is much less prone to outflow obstruction and women rarely need catheterisation for acute retention.

In certain operations, particularly those on the lower abdomen, bladder drainage helps to improve access to the pelvis. A catheter also allows accurate measurement of urine output after major surgery and relieves the immediately postoperative patient from the need to use a urinal.

Intermittent catheterisation, in which a urethral catheter is passed and removed almost immediately, is occasionally necessary as part of a cystometrogram or to administer intravesical drugs. Intermittent catheterisation can be repeated several times a day for patients with chronic urinary retention of neurogenic origin and is usually preferable to an indwelling catheter. Well motivated patients can often be taught to pass the catheter for themselves.

Prolonged catheterisation

Prolonged catheterisation is best avoided. Even with modern anaesthesia, however, a few male patients with retention are unfit for prostatectomy and need an indwelling catheter. Some patients with neurological problems, such as multiple sclerosis, myelodysplasia, or spinal trauma, still require prolonged catheterisation, though most should be treated by means less fraught with long term problems.

151

Catheterisation in the elderly or severely incapacitated incontinent is likewise a measure of final resort.

Contraindications

There are a number of relative contraindications to urethral catheterisation. When urethral injury is suspected after pelvic trauma management of retention is best left in the hands of a urologist. If none is available bladder drainage by a suprapubic catheter is probably safest. Urinary tract infections are very difficult to eradicate in the presence of a catheter, so if a patient has an infection an indwelling catheter should be avoided when possible. When the problem is chronic retention with persistent infection or deteriorating renal function drug treatment, surgical ablation of the sphincters, or intermittent catheterisation should all be considered before long term catheterisation.

Equipment

The procedure requires only the simplest of equipment, but it is infuriating to be gloved and ready to start and then find that something essential is missing. All but the most well organised will find it reassuring to have an assistant ready to run for items which have been forgotten.

In addition to the catheter there should be a tube of local anaesthetic gel, some swabs, and a galley pot of aqueous chlorhexidine on the trolley. Sterile gloves of the cheap polythene variety are perfectly adequate. A single sheet of water repellent paper with a hole cut in the centre is a satisfactory drape. If a self retaining catheter is to be used a syringe filled with sterile water will be needed to inflate the balloon.

When the catheter is inserted it is helpful to have a kidney dish and measuring jug for the urine. If the catheter is to remain in place a drainage bag must also be available. A bag of sterile fluid run through a giving set should be ready to connect to a three way irrigating catheter.

Choice of catheter

Choose the simplest catheter for the job in hand. If the intention is to drain the bladder and then remove the catheter a plain Jaques catheter is enough. A Foley catheter has a balloon which can be inflated to retain it in the bladder. When there is haematuria irrigation can help to prevent clogging of the lumen of the catheter by clots. A three way catheter has an additional channel to run in sterile fluid. A "haematuria" catheter is specially strengthened to stop it collapsing when suction is applied to evacuate clots through it. The most commonly used catheters are shown opposite.

The irritation of the urethra which a catheter causes depends partly upon its chemical composition. A so called "latex" catheter from a reputable manufacturer will have been treated to make it as biologically inert as possible. When

Catheters

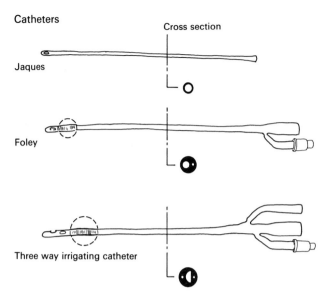

Cross section

Jaques

Foley

Three way irrigating catheter

the catheter is to be in place for more than a few days a silicone one is worth the extra expense.

Finally, there is the question of the correct size of catheter to use. A very large catheter has a tendency to damage the male urethra by causing pressure sores within it. In addition, the paraurethral glands in the bulbar and submeatal regions can be occluded and become infected. This periurethritis seems to predispose to stricture formation. On the other hand, a very fine catheter is easily clogged by blood or debris; also, it will tend to curl in the urethra when it meets an obstruction and is difficult to insert.

It is best to choose a catheter of medium size. These are usually sized using the system invented by Charrière, a Frenchman, and sometimes called French gauge. The Charrière gauge is defined by the circumference of the catheter in millimetres. Since the French, somewhat confusingly, have quite a different sizing system from our own it is probably best to stick to the eponym. A 14 Charrière catheter is a good first choice in the uncomplicated case.

Before you start

Most patients are justifiably alarmed at the thought of being catheterised. Explanation and reassurance are always essential. If a catheter specimen of urine is to be sent for culture the laboratory should be warned that a specimen is on its way.

Procedure

It helps to think of catheterisation in two distinct parts. In the first, local anaesthetic is instilled into the urethra. There must then be a pause of at least five minutes while the

153

anaesthetic works before the second part, the catheterisation itself, can begin. To start catheterising before the anaesthetic works is barbarous. What is more, the urethral sphincter simply reacts to pain by going into spasm and the attempt is very likely to fail.

Instillation of local anaesthetic

It is usual to anaesthetise the urethra with a gel which contains a solution of lignocaine. Some 15–20 ml are instilled, and whether the concentration of lignocaine is 1 or 2% seems to make little difference. Some brands of ligno-caine gel also contain a small concentration of chlorhexidine, though this has not been shown to make any difference to the infection rate after catheterisation.

If care is taken to avoid touching the tip of the nozzle the anaesthetic can be instilled without wearing gloves. When the gel contains antiseptic it is convenient to smear gel around the meatus to create a disinfected field. The nozzle can then be inserted into the urethra through this. The full 15 ml of gel is then squeezed in. If the gel does not contain an antiseptic the skin around the meatus should be disinfected instead with aqueous chlorhexidine on a gauze swab.

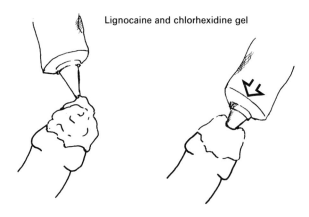
Lignocaine and chlorhexidine gel

In a man, when the anaesthetic gel has been instilled it should be massaged carefully down the urethra to the sphincter. The meatus is squeezed shut and a hand stroked down the anterior surface of the penis. If the patient is cooperative he can hold the tip of his penis betwen finger and thumb to retain the gel in the urethra while it has a chance to work. This is usually more comfortable, convenient, and effective than a mechanical clamp.

It is sometimes said that no local anaesthesia is necessary for catheterisation in women. This is incorrect.

Catheterisation in the male

When five minutes have elapsed since the anaesthetic was instilled catheterisation can begin. With sterile gloves on, swab the penis with antiseptic using a gauze swab. Carefully retract the foreskin, if present, and clean beneath it as well.

Spread the wet swab on the thigh and lay the penis on it while the operating field is covered with the paper sheet. Deliver the penis through the hole in the drape and place the kidney dish close at hand.

Tell the patient that you are about to start. Hold the penis upwards and insert the tip of the catheter into the meatus. The anatomy of the male urethra is shown in the diagram below. There is a small recess in the urethra behind the meatus, but this can be negotiated without difficulty. Pass the catheter gently and deliberately down the urethra until it reaches the penoscrotal junction. Now the tip of the catheter rests against the external urethral sphincter. By pulling the penis downwards between the patient's thighs at this stage, the natural curves of the urethra can be straightened. The axis of the catheter is aligned with the prostatic urethra, and it should advance without difficulty through the sphincter and prostatic urethra and into the bladder.

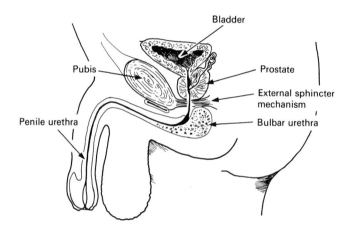

At this stage urine will normally issue from the catheter, showing that it is in the right place. If no urine appears and the catheter seems to be inserted correctly it is worth flushing it with sterile water because the lumen may be blocked by anaesthetic gel. If flushing does not result in a flow of urine it is safest to withdraw the catheter and start again.

When the catheter is clearly in the bladder and urine is coming from it the balloon can be inflated. The volume to be used is marked on the catheter.

When the catheter is safely in place the foreskin must be replaced to avoid the danger of a paraphimosis.

Catheterisation in the female

The female urethra is comparatively short and straight and catheterisation is not usually difficult. The anatomy of the female perineum is shown in the diagram on the following page. The patient should be asked to lie with her thighs apart and her knees comfortably flexed. When the anaesthetic has worked the perineum is swabbed with antiseptic and the field draped with the perforated paper sheet. To reveal the external urethral meatus the labia must first be parted. It lies just posterior to the clitoris and may be surrounded and partly obscured by a frill of soft tissue. Once engaged, the catheter will usually pass without difficulty.

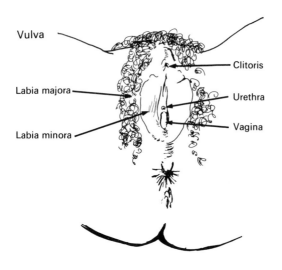

Troubleshooting

If the patient is tense or insufficient time has been allowed for the topical anaesthetic to take effect the catheter may be held up because the urethral sphincter has gone into spasm. If necessary more anaesthetic gel should be instilled and more time given for it to work. Occasionally it is kindest to administer a small dose of benzodiazepine. If the patient is asked to try gently to void when the catheter tip reaches it the sphincter may relax sufficiently to let the catheter through.

If, on the other hand, the urethra is obstructed by a stricture this will usually be apparent because the catheter stops in the penile or bulbar urethra. At the stricture the lumen of the urethra will be reduced to a pinhole and will be surrounded by dense scar tissue. No catheter, however small, will pass until the stricture has been treated by dilation or by urethrotomy. Persisting with the attempt will produce urethral damage. If blood issues from around the catheter it is likely that a false passage is being formed. This is an

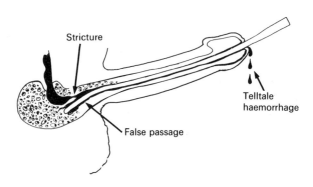

indication to abandon urethral catheterisation and insert a suprapubic catheter instead.

If the prostate is really tight a 14 Charrière catheter may curl up in the urethra and refuse to pass. If this happens it is best to try again, not with a smaller catheter but with a larger one, say 20 Charrière. Larger catheters are rather stiffer and will part the occlusive lobes of the prostate more effectively. They are also blunt ended and less likely to create a false passage. If a larger catheter fails as well it is probably best to get help. If there is a urologist on hand he may well attempt to catheterise the patient using a catheter introducer. This is, however, a dangerous instrument in inexperienced hands because of the ease with which a false passage can be made with it. If in doubt a suprapubic catheter is probably a safer option.

When the balloon of a Foley catheter is blown up the patient should feel no pain. Pain suggests that the balloon is being inflated in the urethra. If this occurs the balloon must be deflated and the catheter repositioned.

Catheterising a female patient is usually easy but problems can arise when there is a variation of the normal anatomy. In some women the urethra is set posteriorly, sometimes actually on the anterior wall of the vagina. In this case exposure may be improved if the patient lies in the left lateral position.

The specimen

It is important to record the volume of urine which is present in the bladder when the catheter is inserted. An aliquot of the urine drained should be sent to the microbiology laboratory without delay.

Aftercare and complications

Short term problems

Many studies have shown that the inevitable onset of infection is delayed if the catheter is connected to a closed drainage bag which is changed each day. If the system has to be opened—for example, to change the bag or to wash out clots occluding the catheter—full sterile precautions are essential. When clots in the bladder are particularly tenacious sterile irrigant flushed down the catheter under pressure will fragment the coagulum so that it can be evacuated in pieces. If clotting is even more troublesome it may be necessary to replace the catheter with one with a larger lumen or with a specially designed haematuria catheter.

Patients who have had chronic retention of urine sometimes have obstructive renal failure. Catheterisation may be followed by a spectacular post-obstructive diuresis with profound metabolic consequences. It is as well to be prepared to put up a drip in these patients since they may not be able to drink enough to keep up with the volumes needed for replacement of their fluid losses.

Long term problems

An indwelling catheter almost always leads to a urinary tract infection within days or weeks. The effects of this can be minimised by regular bladder washouts with saline or dilute chlorhexidine solution. When an infection is established even the most intensive antibiotic treatment is unlikely to make the urine sterile until the catheter is removed. Long term catheterisation with infection is commonly associated with the formation of stones in the bladder.

Irritation of the bladder can produce severe bladder spasms. These are painful and cause bypassing of urine alongside the catheter. Bladder spasms are rarely inhibited by drug treatment, although it is sometimes worth reducing the amount of fluid in the balloon. If there is leakage around the catheter it is futile to put in a larger one. This simply commits the patient to a spiral of increasing catheter size. The urethra becomes steadily more dilated until no catheter can be retained in it.

Frequent washing and the application of antiseptic ointments may inhibit infection, which seems to be associated with the postmeatal strictures that sometimes follow catheterisation. There has been a lot of recent interest in the incidence of strictures after catheterisation. Some are clearly due to faulty technique, but there is evidence that catheters from some manufacturers are more irritant than others. It is probably wise to record the make and even the batch number of each catheter inserted.

Failure of catheter balloon deflation

Beware if the balloon of the catheter fails to deflate when the time comes to remove it. Do not try to burst it by overdistending it. The bladder may burst first. Do not try to instil ether: it can cause a dreadful cystitis. The best way to deal with this problem is to use the fine wire stilette from a ureteric catheter to pass down the inflation channel to burst the balloon. If this fails ultrasound guided percutaneous needle puncture of the balloon is recommended.

Intravenous urography

BENVON CRAMER

GERALD DE LACEY

CAROL RECORD

Introduction

Intravenous urography is an important method of acquiring anatomical information about the urinary tract. In particular it demonstrates the shape and size of the kidneys, calyces, and ureters. However, it provides a crude assessment of renal function which is best assessed with radioisotope studies and measurement of the glomerular filtration rate.

With the increasing availability of ultrasound equipment there are several clinical situations where ultrasonography has replaced intravenous urography. Ultrasound is particularly useful in detecting hydronephrosis and assessing renal shape and size. Similarly, ultrasound has an important role in the follow up of patients with reflux nephropathy and neurological problems affecting bladder function.[1]

Indications

There are several clinical situations where urography is usually the first line imaging procedure. (But remember that in some centres discussion will take place on whether in a particular clinical circumstance another investigation—for example, computed tomography in trauma—might be more appropriate to the particular patient.)

(1) Renal colic or pain relating to the upper renal tract.
(2) Haematuria.
(3) Suspected trauma to the renal tract (urethra excluded).
(4) Demonstration of the course of the ureters prior to surgery for retroperitoneal or pelvic masses.
(5) Infection:
    (a) Suspected tuberculosis of the urinary tract.
    (b) In adults. (In women only if it is a "complicated" infection—for example, associated with loin pain, haematuria, or raised serum creatinine.)[2]
    (c) In infants and children urography is not considered to be a useful first line investigation.[3-4]
(6) Suspected renal mass. It is debatable whether urography or ultrasonography should be the first line investigation. Ultrasonography provides more information on the nature of the mass—for example, whether it is solid or cystic. At present urography is probably the more common request as the first imaging investigation. All the

159

same, strong consideration should be given to selecting ultrasound instead of urography because if a large simple cyst is demonstrated as the cause of the mass then subsequent urography is unnecessary.

Contraindications

No absolute contraindications to urography exist but caution should be observed in five groups.
(1) Patients with known sensitivity to radiological contrast media, patients with asthma, or with a strong history of allergy.
(2) Patients with renal failure: transient rises in serum creatinine after high dose urography have occurred.[5] Care is particularly important in patients with diabetes mellitus and even mild renal failure.[6]
(3) Patients with myeloma.
(4) Neonates.
(5) Pregnant women.

In all these patients careful consideration of the need for intravenous urography is required. Could ultrasonography provide the necessary useful information? If excretion urography is nevertheless regarded as essential then it is important that the patient remains well hydrated both before and after the procedure.

The choice of contrast medium is important. In all these groups the use of the new low osmolar contrast media is recommended.[7] Although they are four to five times as expensive as the standard high osmolar contrast media their use is justified in high risk groups.

Contrast media: suggested doses

Age and indication	Dose	Osmolality
Adults		
Routine	50 ml sodium iothalamate (Conray 420)	High
High risk	70 ml iopamidol (Niopam 300)	Low
Renal failure	2 ml iopamidol (Niopam 300)/kg body weight	Low
Children		
8–12 years	40 ml meglumine iothalamate (Conray 280)	High
4–8 years	20 ml meglumine iothalamate	High
< 4 years	2 ml iopamidol (Niopam 300)/kg to maximum of 20 ml	Low

Note — If a hospital's budget permits, low osmolar contrast media should ideally be used for all intravenous urography. Indeed, this may well become standard practice in the future.

The guidelines for radiographing women of childbearing age have recently been changed. So long as a woman is not pregnant the examination can be performed and need not be restricted to the first 10 days of the menstrual cycle.[8]

Equipment

- Contrast medium (both the standard high osmolar and the more recently introduced low osmolar agents should be available)
- 19 G butterfly needle (smaller gauge for children)
- Syringes (50 and 20 ml)
- Quill
- Injection swabs
- Tape
- Tourniquet
- Compression band
- Vomit bowl
- Emergency drug box with syringes

Drugs to be kept in emergency box

Adrenaline: 1:1000 (1 ml)
Aminophylline: 250 mg in 10 ml
Chlorpheniramine: 10 mg in 1 ml
Frusemide: 20 mg in 2 ml
Hydrocortisone sodium succinate: 100 mg
Water for injection: 2 ml
Metaraminol: 10 mg in 1 ml
Diazepam: 10 mg in 2 ml

Preparation

It is common practice (but not essential) to administer laxatives on the two nights before the procedure. This helps to prevent the kidneys being obscured by faeces. However, some departments do not give laxatives, judging that the slight technical gain is not justified by the expense and the inconvenience to the patient.

Ideally, the patient should remain ambulant for a few hours before the investigation to minimise bowel gas.

There is no indication for dehydration.[9] It can be dangerous and there is little evidence that it improves the urinary concentration of contrast medium.

Some people experience nausea after injection of contrast medium; thus it is advisable to avoid a large meal before the examination.

Inquiry about a history of allergy, asthma, or previous reaction to contrast media is important because all these groups have an increased incidence of reactions.[10] High risk medical groups (patients with myeloma, renal or cardiac failure, diabetes or sickle cell anaemia, and infants and children) should be identified. All these patients should be given a low osmolar contrast medium.

Normal procedure in adults

The basic procedure described here may be modified according to the individual clinical problem.

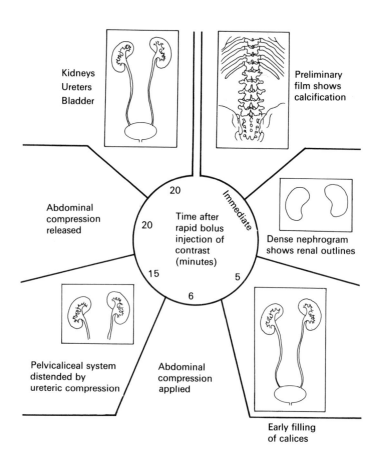

Kidneys
Ureters
Bladder

Preliminary
film shows
calcification

Abdominal
compression
released

Time after
rapid bolus
injection of
contrast
(minutes)

Immediate

20

20

15

6

5

Dense nephrogram
shows renal outlines

Pelvicaliceal system
distended by
ureteric compression

Abdominal
compression
applied

Early filling
of calices

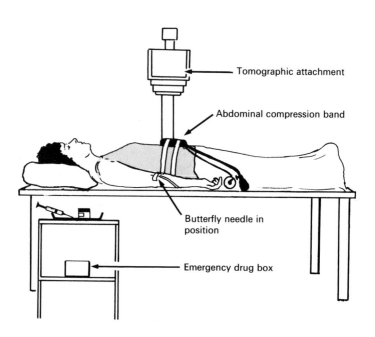

Tomographic attachment

Abdominal compression band

Butterfly needle in
position

Emergency drug box

Immediately before the investigation the patient empties the bladder. A control abdominal film is taken to show renal tract calcification. With the patient supine, contrast is injected rapidly as a bolus through a butterfly needle preferably sited in the median antecubital vein. Rapid injection is required to obtain the high serum concentration necessary for a dense nephrogram (the radiographic image of the renal parenchyma shown on the film taken immediately after the injection).

Film sequence

(1) An *immediate* post-injection film of the renal areas to show the outlines of the kidneys.

(2) A *five minute* film of the renal tract to assess distension of the calyces and to demonstrate the distal ureters before they are obscured by a contrast filled bladder.

(3) Application of an abdominal compression band to distend the upper tracts unless there is a contraindication, such as:

   (a) the five minute film has shown distension of the calyces;

   (b) renal colic;

   (c) after trauma;

   (d) recent abdominal surgery;

   (e) a large abdominal mass.

   A *15 minute* film of the renal area to show the distended pelvicalyceal systems.

(4) At *20 minutes*, following release of the compression band, an abdominal film to show the ureters and bladder.

(5) A *post-micturition* bladder film is probably only indicated in haematuria, suspected urethral diverticulum in women, and vesicoureteric calculi.[11-12] Post-micturition residue in males can usually be demonstrated on the control film[11] and thus even in prostatism it is not really necessary to obtain this additional film of the bladder.

Modifications

(1) For *children and infants* a different approach is required. The volume of contrast is reduced in relation to body weight. The number of exposures is reduced to a minimum and gonad protection is used whenever possible. A fizzy drink may produce a gas filled stomach, which acts as a window through which to view the kidneys. In children aged under 4 a low osmolar contrast medium is recommended and should be injected slowly. A control film and films of the renal area at the end of injection and of the abdomen at 10 minutes are usually sufficient. Compression is not required.

(2) In *renal colic* a preliminary film and a seven minute film are often sufficient to confirm or exclude the diagnosis.

(3) In *renal failure* (Are you sure an ultrasound examination has not provided all the useful clinical information?) a low osmolar contrast medium is chosen and the maxi-

mum possible dose of contrast is injected (600 mg I_2/kg). Tomography will help to delineate poorly opacified calyces and renal parenchyma.

Troubleshooting

To recognise complications and deal with them promptly it is advisable to leave the butterfly needle in situ until the examination is complete. The patient should not be left unattended during the 20 minutes after injection.

Patients with a history of allergy, asthma, or previous reaction to contrast warrant low osmolar contrast media. But even before proceeding to urography, strong consideration should be given to whether ultrasound is all that might be needed. Should urography be deemed necessary, pretreatment with steroids (for example, in the 18 hours before the investigation) should be considered in those with a previous contrast reaction, as there is some evidence that this reduces the incidence of adverse reactions.[7,13–15]

High risk groups merit the low osmolar contrast media. Low osmolar contrast media are more physiological and result in less tissue toxicity, less haemodynamic disturbance, and fewer severe reactions. However, because of the high cost of the low osmolar media, it remains common practice in many hospitals for the cheaper high osmolar media to be used for all other patients. Remember, *never* dehydrate patients in the high risk medical groups.

Complications and aftercare

Some patients will experience minor unpleasant sensations after intravenous injection of contrast—nausea, warmth, metallic taste, shivering, and sneezing. Reassurance is all that is required. Minor reactions may be either allergic or idiosyncratic and include urticaria, rhinitis, and conjunctivitis. In most instances reassurance will suffice. If severe, antihistamines may be needed. Chlorpheniramine maleate 10–20 mg intravenously usually induces a rapid symptomatic response. Bronchospasm may occur and can be quite severe, especially in known asthmatics. Oxygen, aminophylline 250 mg given intravenously over five minutes, and hydrocortisone sodium succinate 100–400 mg intravenously may be required.

Acute anaphylaxis is manifested by urticaria, bronchospasm, glottic and angioneurotic oedema and may lead to circulatory collapse and pulmonary oedema. In addition to oxygen, hydrocortisone, and antihistamines, 0·5–1·0 ml of adrenaline 1:1000 subcutaneously may be required. In life threatening situations a tracheostomy or cricothyroid puncture will be necessary.

Vasovagal reactions and cardiac arrest can also occur. For 40 000 procedures involving contrast media there are 2500–4000 adverse reactions, 50–80 serious reactions, and one death. The *x* ray department must always have facilities and a protocol available for immediate resuscitation.

Regarding aftercare, the main concern is to encourage fluids to prevent dehydration. This is particularly important in high risk patients with renal impairment, diabetes mellitus, or myeloma, because the combination of intravascular contrast medium and dehydration can exacerbate or precipitate renal failure.[6]

Interpretation of results

The control film is assessed for the presence of calcification related to the urinary tract. Is there generalised or localised calcification in the kidneys? Is there calcification in the line of the ureters or bladder? The relationship of the calcification to anatomical structures—for example, the calyces or renal artery—or "tumours" will become clearer on subsequent films.

Residual bladder volume can be shown on the control abdominal radiograph.

The nephrogram is shown on the films taken immediately after injection of contrast and will show the position, size, and shape of the kidneys. The outlines are assessed for scarring, enlargement, or the presence of a "filling defect" caused by a "tumour."

The later films will show the pelvicalyceal systems, ureters, and bladder. The important features to look for are dilatation, both localised and generalised, persistent narrowing, distortion, deviation, and delayed or incomplete filling of the collecting systems.

In the absence of a pyelogram (contrast filled pelvicalyceal system) a nephrogram may persist and its behaviour is helpful in determining the aetiology. If both kidneys are affected then a low urinary tract obstruction or a generalised disorder affecting both kidneys is likely.

The bladder outline is inspected for diverticula, trabeculation, and an elevated base due to prostatic hypertrophy. Filling defects may be outlined more clearly on a film taken after micturition.

1 Brandt TD, Neiman HL, Calenoff L, Greenberg M, Kaplan PE, Nanninga JB. Ultrasound evaluation of the urinary system in spinal cord-injury patients. *Radiology* 1981;**141**:473–7.
2 De Lange EE, Jones B. Unnecessary intravenous urography in young women with recurrent urinary tract infections. *Clin Rad* 1983;**34**:551–3.
3 Whitaker RH, Sherwood T. Another look at diagnostic pathways in children with urinary tract infection. *Br Med J* 1984;**288**:839–41.
4 Sherwood T, Whitaker RH. Initial screening of children with urinary tract infections: is plain film radiography and ultrasonography enough? *Br Med J* 1984;**288**:827.
5 Webb JAW, Reznek RH, Cattell WR, Kelsey Fry I. Renal function after high dose urography in patients with renal failure. *Br J Rad* 1981;**54**:479–83.
6 Byrd L, Sherman RL. Radio contrast-induced acute renal failure: a clinical and pathophysiologic review. *Medicine (Baltimore)* 1979;**58**:270–9.

7 Grainger RG. The clinical and financial implications of the low-osmolar radiological contrast media. (Letter) *Clin Rad* 1984;**35**:251–2.

8 National Radiological Protection Board. Exposure to ionising radiation of pregnant women. Advice on the diagnostic exposure of women who are, or who may be, pregnant. London: HMSO, March 1985. (ASP8.)

9 Bell KE, McIlrath EM. Dehydration in urography: is it really necessary? *Clin Rad* 1985;**36**:311–12.

10 Ansell G, Tweedie MCK, West CR, Price Evans DA, Couch L. The current status of reactions to intravenous contrast media. *Invest Radiol* 1980;**15**(suppl);32–9.

11 Morewood DJW, Scally JK. An evaluation of the post-micturition radiograph following intravenous urography. *Clin Rad* 1986;**37**:499–500.

12 Gerber WL, Brown RC. The value of post-void radiographs in excretory urography. *Clin Rad* 1985;**36**:525–7.

13 Lasser EC, Lang J, Sovak M, Kolb W, Lyon S, Hamlin AE. Steroids: theoretical and experimental basis for utilization in prevention of contrast media reactions. *Radiology* 1977;**125**:1–9.

14 Rapoport S, Bookstein JJ, Higgins CB, Carey PH, Sovak M, Lasser EC. Experience with metrizamide in patients with previous severe anaphylactoid reactions to ionic contrast agents. *Radiology* 1982;**143**:321–5.

15 Lasser EC, Berry CC, Talner LB, Santini LC, Lang EK, Gerber FH, Stolberg HO. Pretreatment with corticosteroids to alleviate reactions to intravenous contrast material. *N Engl J Med* 1987;**317**:845–9.

Prostatic biopsy

J R RHIND

Introduction

The diagnosis of adenocarcinoma of the prostate based solely on digital examination of the gland will be correct in only 50% of cases. Prostatic calculi, the fibrous prostate, granulomatous prostatitis, sarcoma, and transitional carcinomatous infiltration may each cause the prostate to feel firmer than normal.

Oestrogens or orchidectomy will be of no benefit in these conditions and may cause harm. Histological or cytological proof of the diagnosis is essential.

Examination of prostatic tissue obtained by biopsy has been used to assess the response of a tumour to either hormonal or cytotoxic manipulation or radiotherapy. Biopsy tissue examined bacteriologically may also be helpful in prostatitis.

Open biopsy of the prostate by either the perineal or retropubic route is rarely used in the United Kingdom. Although the open approach allows the surgeon the greatest accuracy in obtaining a specimen from a suspicious nodule, there is a greatly increased morbidity. There is also the risk that resulting fibrosis might make later total prostatectomy or cystoprostatectomy more difficult and that there may be wound seeding with malignancy.

Aspiration of the prostate using the Franzen needle to obtain cells for cytology is the most innocuous form of biopsy but, unfortunately, requires the services of a pathologist who is familiar with prostatic cytology and is therefore not always possible.

The most common method of biopsy is the punch or needle method using the Tru-Cut needle or the Franklin modification of the Vim–Silverman needle. This provides a core of tissue suitable for routine histological examination.

Contraindications

Contraindications to prostatic biopsy are few. Since the procedure can be performed in the lateral position with any degree of tilt necessary to the patient even the most severely orthopnoeic can be managed. The common blood clotting disorders can be easily dealt with and the only caveat would be the patient with unsuspected marrow involvement by malignancy. It would, in such cases, probably be wiser to use the rectal route so that direct finger pressure on the biopsy site can be applied should excess bleeding occur.

Equipment

The equipment necessary is very little. Apart from the Tru-Cut needle and a pair of rubber gloves, some skin cleanser and a size 15 blade will be required if the perineal route is to be used.

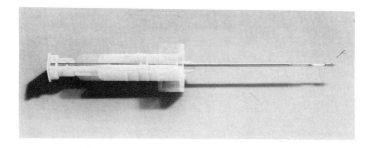

Procedure

Needle biopsy may be performed as a day case procedure, but since penetration of the prostate by the needle causes some discomfort general anaesthesia, local block, or intra-muscular pethidine and diazepam are necessary. The patient is placed in either the lithotomy or lateral position with any degree of Trendelenburg thought to be necessary. Very few patients are unsuitable because of ill health or inaccessibility of the prostate.

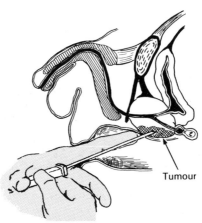

Tumour

The biopsy may be performed using either a perineal or transrectal route.

(1) *Perineal route*—Sampling via the perineal route is a semisterile technique and requires the perineum to be shaved and the skin cleansed in the usual manner. A tiny incision in the midline is made with a size 15 blade

1·0–1·5 cm anterior to the anal verge. The biopsy needle is inserted through this incision into the prostate and its course to the area to be sampled estimated by placing a finger in the rectum.

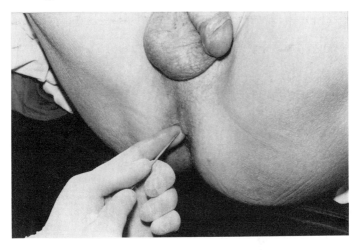

(2) *Transrectal route*—Transrectal biopsy entails passing the needle with the examining finger into the rectum and is therefore a non-sterile technique. To minimise trauma to the anal mucosa the sharp tip of the needle should be protected by the pulp of the finger during insertion. The surgeon then palpates the area of prostate in doubt and the needle is introduced direct through the rectal mucosa.

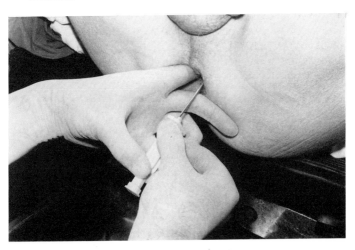

In both methods tissue is obtained by advancing the trocar and then closing the cannula onto the trocar. With a little practice the trocar may be held firmly by the remaining fingers of the left hand so that removal of the finger from the rectum is not necessary. The tissue is then placed in preservative for histological examination or transport medium for bacteriological examination. Several samples may be obtained at the same time, although this slightly increases the risk of complications.

The specimen

The specimen is placed in formalin solution for histological examination and normal saline if for bacteriology. Remember to note on the form if the patient has already received irradiation, chemotherapy, or immunotherapy since ignorance of these facts may make interpretation much more difficult for the histologist.

Complications

Biopsy failure occurs when no tissue is obtained or the histology of the specimen does not agree with the final diagnosis. The transrectal route has a lower failure rate than the perineal one. This is partly because the operator has a better idea of which portion of the prostate the needle is sampling, but also because carcinoma tends to arise in the peripheral part of the gland. This area may be missed when the perineal route is used, although with practice the accuracy of this method should improve. Biopsy failure may also occur when the patient has had a prostatectomy so that only the relatively thin shell of the false capsule remains, or when the tissue is so friable that none can be picked up by the needle.

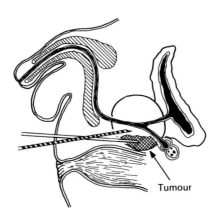

Tumour

Rectal bleeding or haematuria may occur after biopsy but is only rarely a problem. Haematuria is not uncommon when biopsy is by the perineal route and may persist for several days, but unless the patient has coagulation problems transfusion is unnecessary.

Infection shown as pyrexia after using the transrectal route may develop in up to 25% of cases and may proceed to bacteriogenic shock. It is now recommended that prophylactic trimethoprim be given to cover the procedure.

Tumour implantation is the fear in any biopsy procedure but is extremely rare in the case of prostatic needle biopsy and has been reported only in association with the perineal route.

Vaginal examination and taking a smear

ELIZABETH FORSYTHE

Introduction

A vaginal examination includes inspection of the external genitalia, a bimanual digital examination, and an internal examination of the vagina using a speculum. It should always be preceded by an abdominal examination. If the examination is done with sensitivity on the part of the doctor and with the full cooperation of the patient it can help with the diagnosis of not only physical problems but also psychological and sexual ones.

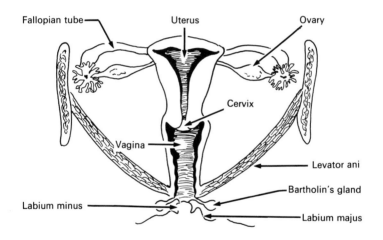

Indications

(1) A screening procedure including the taking of a smear.
(2) Part of a general gynaecological examination to investigate gynaecological signs and symptoms.
(3) Obstetric management.
(4) Investigation of a genitourinary problem.
(5) In the family planning consultation for excluding gynaecological disease, before fitting an intrauterine contraceptive device or a diaphragm, or in the investigation and treatment of a psychosexual problem.

(6) The investigation of wider clinical problems including lower abdominal pain, endocrinological abnormalities, or lower limb oedema.

Contraindications

Possibly the procedure is contraindicated for the virgin of any age; but if the patient is relaxed and there is good communication between the doctor and the patient examination may be possible with one finger and the use of a very small speculum.

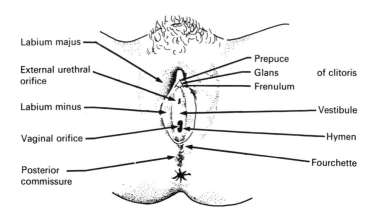

The vulva of a virgin.

Equipment

- An examination room screened from sight and if possible from sound
- A standard bench type couch with a waterproof covering and disposable paper coverings
- An efficient adjustable light
- Disposable plastic gloves
- K-Y or other lubricating jelly
- A variety of sizes of bivalve speculae including one suitable for the examination of a virgin
- A Sims speculum
- Swabs, forceps for holding a sponge, and long Spencer–Wells forceps
- A clean towel or sheet for covering the patient's abdomen and thighs
- Tampons and sanitary pads
- For taking a smear: glass slides, a pencil for writing the patient's name, a choice of spatulas, fixative, and a slide holder for transport
- For taking swabs: sterile swabs and transport media for bacteria and viruses as supplied by the laboratory

- The correct forms for sending with the specimens
- A microscope for the immediate diagnosis of trichomonas
  Note—All instruments should be autoclaved.

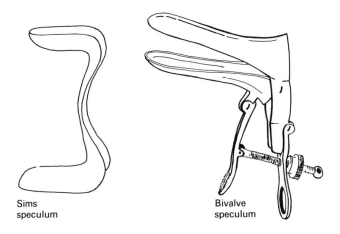

Sims speculum

Bivalve speculum

Before you start

The laboratory should be alerted if results are required urgently. The investigation of chlamydia and herpes needs rapid transport to the laboratory—certainly within 24 hours.

Check that the patient has emptied her bladder, unless she is being examined for prolapse or stress incontinence. Arrange for the collection of a midstream specimen of urine, if necessary.

Before taking a smear check that the patient has not had sexual intercourse in the previous 24 hours and has not inserted a diaphragm.

Procedure

A male doctor usually prefers to have a chaperone present. It is important that the doctor talks to the patient during the examination, explains what he is doing, and remains aware of the patient's feelings.

Plastic gloves must be worn on both hands.

The dorsal position is the most commonly used. The patient lies on her back with her knees flexed and her hips flexed and abducted. Her abdomen and thighs should be covered so that she feels less exposed. Raising the head of the couch makes the patient more comfortable and helps her to relax. She will be able to see what the doctor is doing and may be less apprehensive. However, she may prefer to be in the position in which she has been examined previously.

The left lateral position is useful for the woman with reduced mobility of her hips and the very embarrassed patient. It gives good exposure of the anus, perineum, and the posterior parts of the vulva and is useful for examining, with the Sims speculum, a prolapse in an obese patient.

173

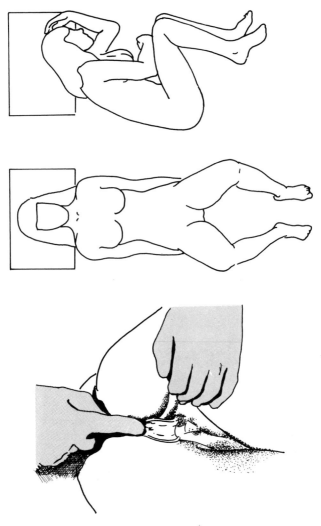

Insertion of Sims speculum.

It is helpful to make physical contact with the patient while you explain the procedure to her—for example, if she is in the dorsal position your left hand could be rested against her right knee. If she shows distress at any time during the examination you must discover whether it is because of pain, fear, her embarrassment, your embarrassment, or your clumsiness. The examination follows a sequence from external genitalia, vagina, cervix, uterus, adnexae, and pouch of Douglas.

External inspection

Notice if there is a smell—for example, the bad smell of a retained tampon. Inspect the urethral opening for a discharge, urethritis, or a caruncle. Ask the patient to cough and observe if there is any leakage of urine and to push down to look for any prolapse. Note also any vaginal discharge, the state of the skin, the presence of an intact hymen, ulceration, tumour, warts, or herpes. Take swabs if necessary.

174

Internal inspection

This should be done before bimanual digital examination if a smear is to be taken. The size of the speculum used will depend on the patient's menstrual, sexual, and obstetric history. If the internal inspection of a virgin is to be attempted choose a very small speculum. Warm the speculum in warm water and check the temperature against your gloved hand before use. No lubricant apart from water should be used when taking a smear.

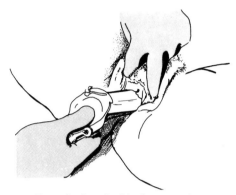

Introducing the bivalve speculum.

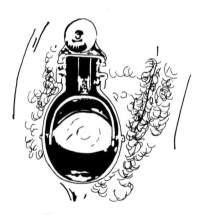

Exposure of cervix.

While standing at the right of the patient hold the speculum in the right hand and with the left hand gently separate the labia minora. The speculum can be introduced with the blades vertical or at an angle of 45° from the vertical. As the blades enter the vagina rotate them until they are horizontal, exerting gentle pressure against the posterior wall of the vagina. Observing the direction of the vagina, push the speculum upwards and backwards until the blades can be opened to expose the cervix. Difficulty in exposing the cervix may be due to using too large or too short a speculum, the speculum being too far anterior or posterior, or to vaginismus. Note the size, shape, and appearance of the cervix. Is there ulceration, erosion, a polyp, tear, or discharge?

Taking a smear—Have the marked slide and fixative ready. The cells to be examined must come from the squamocolumnar junction, which may be inside the cervical canal. Good exposure of the cervix is vital. Insert the forked end of a wooden or plastic spatula into the cervical canal and rotate it through 360°. Exert enough pressure to sample the cells, but do not press hard enough to cause bleeding. Spread the material thinly on the slide. Spray immediately with fixative or immerse in fixative. After 10 to 15 minutes drain off surplus fixative and put the slide in a transporter.

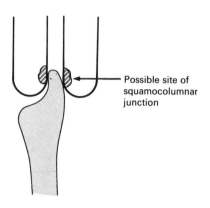

Possible site of squamocolumnar junction

Taking a swab—For ulcers use a dry sterile swab and swab firmly from the base of the lesion. For chlamydia and mycoplasma swab from around the cervix and into the endocervical canal. For vaginal discharge take a swab from high up in the posterior fornix. Break the end of the swab off and place it in the appropriate medium. Refrigerate if necessary. Arrange transport.

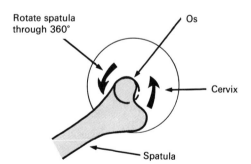

Rotate spatula through 360°

Os

Cervix

Spatula

The blades of the speculum must be opened slightly before its withdrawal. But do not catch the cervix between the blades; this is uncomfortable for the patient. The walls of the vagina can best be observed during removal of the speculum. Any discharge or surplus lubricant left on the vulva should be gently wiped away with a swab. If necessary the patient should be given a tampon or pad.

Bimanual digital examination

This can be done before internal inspection if you are not taking a smear. Insert the well lubricated index finger of the right hand (some doctors use two fingers but this is more uncomfortable and seldom necessary) into the vagina while separating the labia minora with the left. The left hand is then placed on the abdomen below the umbilicus and moved slowly downwards. The hand on the abdomen is more effective for feeling the pelvic organs than the finger(s) in the vagina. The finger in the anterior fornix pushes the cervix as far backwards as possible. The uterus can then be brought forwards and palpated between the right finger and the left hand. Its size, shape, position, and mobility can be estimated.

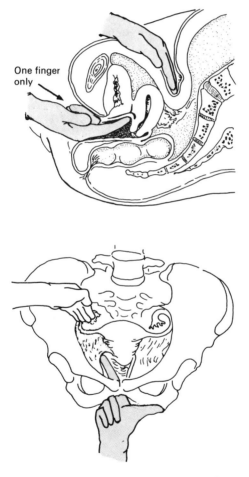

The examining finger is moved towards one fornix and the hand on the abdomen is moved to the same side. The ovary may be felt; the normal ovary is tender when palpated bimanually. The normal fallopian tube is not palpable. The other lateral fornix is checked and the finger is moved into the posterior fornix to examine the pouch of Douglas. The finger is examined for blood and discharge when it is withdrawn. If a vaginal examination is impossible a rectal one may be done.

Troubleshooting

Vaginismus, a tightening of the levator muscles, can make the use of a speculum impossible—for example, it may not be possible to enter the vagina, or tightening of the muscles after the speculum is in position may cause the patient considerable pain. Do not proceed with the examination if it is painful. Try to understand the reason for the difficulty.

The specimen

Smears should be fixed with the fluid available—usually equal parts of absolute alcohol and methylated ether. Transport medium for swabs is supplied by the laboratory and must be stored at the recommended temperature. A culture plate may be used for the investigation of gonorrhoea.

Labelling

The date and time that the specimens were taken must be written both on the form and the specimen. On the form write details about the patient, the identity of the specimen, from where it was collected, the clinical details, and which antibiotics have been given and when.

Aftercare

When the patient is dressed it is advisable to discuss the clinical findings with her and tell her what tests are being done, how long the results will be, and the arrangements for follow up.

Interpretation of results

When the results of a cervical smear test will be available depends on the local cytology service. Usually swab results will be available in a week but some, such as actinomycosis, will take much longer.

Index